Contents

THE Diabetes

Your Complete Exercise Guide

The Cooper Clinic and Research Institute Fitness Series

Neil F. Gordon, MD, PhD, MPH
The Cooper Institute for Aerobics Research
Dallas, Texas

Human Kinetics Publishers

In memory of Marilyn Martens,
cofounder of Human Kinetics Publishers,
who fought a long and courageous battle with the complications of diabetes.

Library of Congress Cataloging-in-Publication Data

Gordon, Neil F.
    Diabetes : your complete exercise guide / Neil F. Gordon.
      p.   cm.
    Includes index.
    ISBN 0-87322-427-2
      1. Diabetes--Exercise therapy.   I. Title.
    RC661.E94G67   1993
    616.4'62062--dc20

ACCN.   B29044

I. Title.   616.462

T.   92-39741
             CIP

ISBN: 0-87322-427-2

Notice: Exercise and health are matters that vary necessarily between individuals. Readers should speak with their own doctors about their individual needs *before* starting any exercise program. This book is *not* intended as a substitute for the medical advice and supervision of your personal physician. Any application of the recommendations set forth in the following pages is at the reader's discretion and sole risk.

Human Kinetics books are available at special discounts for bulk purchase. Special editions or book excerpts can also be created to specification. For details, contact the Special Sales Manager at Human Kinetics.

Printed in the United States of America   10 9 8 7 6 5 4

Human Kinetics
Web site: http://www.humankinetics.com

United States: Human Kinetics
P.O. Box 5076, Champaign, IL 61825-5076
1-800-747-4457

Canada: Human Kinetics, Box 24040, Windsor, ON N8Y 4Y9
1-800-465-7301 (in Canada only)

Europe: Human Kinetics, P.O. Box IW14
Leeds LS16 6TR, United Kingdom
(44) 1132 781708

Australia: Human Kinetics, 57A Price Avenue
Lower Mitcham, South Australia 5062
(08) 277 1555

New Zealand: Human Kinetics, P.O. Box 105-231, Auckland 1
(09) 523 3462

Foreword

This is one in a series of five books, each of which covers an exercise rehabilitation program we at the Cooper Clinic and Research Institute devised to help our patients and others around the world recover from the chronic disorders of arthritis, chronic fatigue, breathing problems, stroke, and diabetes. You hold the diabetes book in your hand.

Diabetes is widespread, ranking as one of the most common chronic diseases. In the United States, 10 million people have non-insulin-dependent, or Type II, diabetes, and as many as 1 million others are thought to have insulin-dependent (Type I) diabetes. Collectively, they make up almost 5% of the U.S. population. This book is addressed to those 11 million people, and others like them around the world, who have been living with diabetes for months, maybe years. From our experiences with diabetes patients at the Cooper Clinic and Research Institute, we know such people can benefit greatly from the lifestyle approach to total well-being that we advocate. What's the lifestyle approach? It's a combination of regular aerobic and other forms of exercise, good nutrition, and a balanced, moderate outlook on modern life with its many tensions and stresses. As a diabetes patient, you need to realize that medication alone is not what your rehabilitation is all about. Insulin and other drugs, although vitally important, are not enough to make people with diabetes feel great and live full lives.

The components of diabetes treatment and rehabilitation are represented visually in Figure 1. These interlocking circles represent the symbolic balance between the mainstays of diabetes management: diet, exercise, and insulin. It is because exercise is not emphasized enough in the many diabetes treatment books already on the market that we felt it necessary to write this one.

What this book offers that most others don't is comprehensive, state-of-the-art advice on how a diabetes patient should go about starting a regular exercise program, including essential information about just how much exercise you need to do to improve your health. Furthermore, in this book, we'll show you precisely how regular exercise fits into a comprehensive diabetes treatment and rehabilitation program. We'll educate you about exercise's benefits as well as its potential risks. And we'll offer sensible, easy-to-follow guidelines for juggling the constraints of insulin and other drug therapy with the physical demands that exercise places on the body.

At the Cooper Clinic and Research Institute, it's our hope that this book will serve as a springboard for discussions about exercise between you and your doctor or the other members of your diabetes health-care team—your nurse educator and dietitian, for example. We also hope it will make you more self-sufficient and less dependent on your health-care team for all the details on how to work exercise into your daily routine. On the other hand, we don't ever want you to regard our advice as a substitute for that of your physician or other team members.

Make no mistake about it. Diabetes is more complicated than many diseases. This, in fact, is probably why many diabetes patients aren't

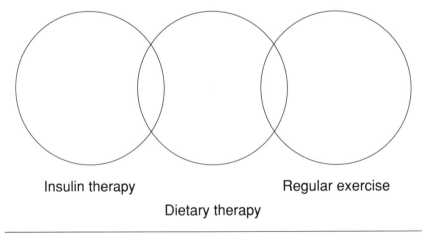

Insulin therapy   Regular exercise

Dietary therapy

Figure 1.   Three major factors in the management of diabetes.

better informed about their illness and how regular exercise fits into the picture. There are real physical payoffs that people with diabetes can derive from exercise, and this book will tell you about them.

Readers familiar with my books know that I believe people need all the motivation they can get to break a bad health habit and replace it with a good one. To provide you, the diabetes patient, with a strong incentive to maintain your health through regular exertion (while preventing an exercise-induced blood-sugar emergency), this book comes complete with a Health Points System. It's a great system designed to keep you exercising over the long haul. It will ease you into a healthier lifestyle and motivate you to keep going and persevere even on those days when you feel most tempted to backslide.

The Cooper Clinic and Research Institute Fitness Series is directed at people who have been diagnosed with a serious medical problem and want to do something about it. I anticipate that the readers of these rehabilitation books will be highly motivated fighters, people who aren't going to let a chronic illness or disorder get the best of them. They're going to do what needs to be done to fight back and win!

If you're a fighter and a winner, you've got the right book in your hands, for I believe my staff at The Cooper Aerobics Center* and I have developed one of America's finest diabetes rehabilitation programs. A safe exercise regimen is the foundation of that program.

I want you to do more than just fill your head with the medical and exercise facts contained in this book. I urge you to act on what you learn. You might want to think of *Diabetes: Your Complete Exercise Guide* as a means to two very worthwhile ends: prolonging your life and improving the quality of your added months and years. By working closely with your own physician and adhering to our program, you stand the best chance of all of improving both the quality and quantity of your years. Good luck. And the best of health to you!

Kenneth H. Cooper, MD, MPH

---

*The Cooper Aerobics Center, founded by Ken Cooper in Dallas in the early 1970s, is comprised of the Cooper Clinic, a preventive and rehabilitative medicine facility; The Cooper Institute for Aerobics Research, where researchers study the role of exercise and other lifestyle factors in the maintenance of health; the Cooper Wellness Program, which provides a supportive, live-in environment where participants can focus time and attention on the challenging task of how to make positive lifestyle changes; and the Cooper Fitness Center, a health club in which all members' exercise efforts are supervised by a well-trained staff of health professionals.

About the Author

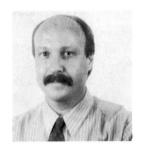

D r. Neil F. Gordon is widely regarded as a leading medical authority on exercise and health. Before receiving his master's degree in public health from the University of California at Los Angeles in 1989, Dr. Gordon received doctoral degrees in exercise physiology and medicine at the University of the Witwatersrand in Johannesburg, South Africa. He also served as medical director of cardiac rehabilitation and exercise physiology for 6 years at I Military Hospital in Pretoria, South Africa.

Since 1987, Dr. Gordon has been the director of exercise physiology at the internationally renowned Cooper Institute for Aerobics Research in Dallas, Texas. He has written over 50 papers related to exercise and medicine. Dr. Gordon is also coauthor of the book *Don't Count Yourself Out: Staying Fit after Thirty-Five with Jimmy Connors*.

Dr. Gordon is a member of the American Heart Association and American Diabetes Association. He is a fellow of the American College of Sports Medicine and the American Association of Cardiovascular and Pulmonary Rehabilitation. He also has served on the boards of directors for AACVPR, the Texas Association of Cardiovascular and Pulmonary Rehabilitation, and the American Heart Association (Dallas affiliate).

Preface

Any series of books as comprehensive as The Cooper Clinic and Research Institute Fitness Series is likely to have an interesting story behind it, and this one certainly does. The story began over a decade ago, shortly after I completed my medical training. Because of my keen interest in sports medicine (which was why I went to medical school in the first place), I volunteered to help establish an exercise rehabilitation program for patients with chronic diseases at a major South African hospital. To get the ball rolling I decided to telephone patients who had recently been treated at the hospital. My very first call planted the seed for writing a series of books that would (a) educate patients with chronic medical conditions about the many benefits of a physically active lifestyle and (b) lead them step-by-step down the road to improved health.

That telephone call was an eye-opener for me, a relative novice in the field of rehabilitation medicine. The patient, a middle-aged man who had recently suffered a heart attack, bellowed into the phone: "Why are you trying to create more problems for me? Isn't it enough that I've been turned into an invalid for the rest of my life by a heart attack?" Fortunately, I kept my cool and convinced him to give the program a try—after all, what did he have to lose? Within months he was "miraculously" transformed into a man with a new zest for life. Like the thousands of men and women with chronic disorders with whom I've subsequently worked in South Africa and, more recently, the United States, he had experienced first-hand the numerous physical and psychological benefits of a medically prescribed exercise rehabilitation program.

Today it's known that a comprehensive exercise rehabilitation program, such as the one outlined in this book, is an essential component of state-of-the-art medical care for patients with a variety of chronic conditions, including diabetes. But, despite the many benefits unfolding through numerous research studies, patients with chronic medical conditions are usually not much better informed than that heart patient was prior to my telephone call. This book is meant to help fill this void for persons with diabetes by providing you with practical, easy-to-follow information about exercise rehabilitation for use in collaboration with your doctor.

To accomplish this, I've set up this book as follows. In chapter 1 you'll meet two of our diabetes patients, whose stories will introduce you to some basic truths about diabetes, exercise, and rehabilitation. In chapter 2 you'll discover the wonderful benefits of a physically active lifestyle. Toward the end of this chapter, however, I try to temper my obvious enthusiasm for exercise by pointing out some of its potential risks for persons with diabetes. In chapter 3 I show you step-by-step how to embark on a sensible exercise rehabilitation program. In chapter 4 you'll learn how to use the Health Points System to determine precisely how much exercise you need to do to optimize your health and fitness, without exerting yourself to the point where exercise can become risky. At the end of this chapter, I'll give you some useful tips for sticking with your exercise program once you get started. In chapter 5 I share with you the steps you should take to prevent a blood-sugar emergency during or after exercise. Finally, in chapter 6 I provide you with more essential safety guidelines. Although exercise is a far more normal state for the human body than being sedentary, I want you to keep your risk, however small it may be, as low as possible.

When using the programs in this book, please view them as a blueprint and be sure the aims you set for yourself are realistic. It is up to you and your doctor to make changes in this blueprint; that is, to adapt my programs to suit your medical condition. Above all, remember that no book can remove the need for close supervision by a patient's own doctor.

I hope that when you finish reading this book, you'll have new hope for a healthier, longer, more enjoyable life. If you then act on my advice and adopt a more physically active lifestyle, this book will have supplemented the efforts of the American Diabetes Association and other similar organizations around the world in the battle against diabetes. If it does, the many hours spent preparing *Diabetes: Your Complete Exercise Guide* will have been well worth the effort.

Neil F. Gordon, MD, PhD, MPH

Acknowledgments

To prepare a series of books as comprehensive and complex as this, I have required the assistance and cooperation of many talented people. To adequately acknowledge all would be impossible. However, I would be remiss not to recognize a few special contributions.

Ken Cooper, MD, MPH, chairman and founder of the Cooper Clinic, was of immense assistance in initiating this series. In addition to writing the foreword and providing many useful suggestions, he continues to serve as an inspiration to me and millions of people around the world.

Larry Gibbons, MD, MPH, medical director of the Cooper Clinic, coauthored with me *The Cooper Clinic Cardiac Rehabilitation Program*. In doing so he made an invaluable contribution to many of the concepts used in this series, especially the Health Points System.

Jacqueline Thompson, a talented writer based in Staten Island, New York, provided excellent editorial assistance with the first draft of this series. Her contributions and those of Herb Katz, a New York-based literary agent, greatly enhanced the practical value of this series.

Charles Sterling, EdD, executive director of The Cooper Institute for Aerobics Research, provided much needed guidance and support while working on this series. So too did John Duncan, PhD; Chris Scott, MS; Pat Brill, PhD; Kia Vaandrager, MS; Conrad Earnest, MS;

Sheila Burford; and my many other colleagues at the Institute, Cooper Clinic, Cooper Wellness Program, and Cooper Fitness Center.

Edward Horton, MD, a world-renowned diabetes authority from the Joslin Diabetes Center, Harvard Medical School, Boston, reviewed the first draft of *Diabetes: Your Complete Exercise Guide* and provided many excellent suggestions.

My thanks to Rainer Martens, president of Human Kinetics Publishers, without whom this series could not have been published. Rainer, Holly Gilly (my developmental editor), and other staff members at Human Kinetics Publishers did a fantastic job in making this series a reality. It was a pleasurable and gratifying experience to work with them.

A special thanks to the patients who allowed me to tell their stories and to all my patients over the years from whom I have learned so much about exercise and rehabilitation.

Finally I want to thank my wonderful family—my wife, Tracey, and daughters, Kim and Terri—for their patience, support, and understanding in preparing this series.

To these people and the many others far too numerous to list, many thanks for making this book a reality and in so doing benefiting patients with diabetes around the world.

Credits

Developmental Editor—Holly Gilly; *Assistant Editors*—Valerie Hall, Julie Swadener, John Wentworth; *Copyeditor*—Jane Bowers; *Proofreader*—Karin Leszczynski; *Indexer*—Sheila Ary; *Production Director*—Ernie Noa; *Text Design*—Keith Blomberg; *Text Layout*—Sandra Meier, Tara Welsch; *Cover Design*—Jack Davis; *Factoids*—Doug Burnett; *Technique Drawings*—Tim Offenstein; *Interior Art*—Kathy Fuoss, Gretchen Walters; *Printer*—United Graphics

The Cooper Clinic and Research Institute Fitness Series

Arthritis: *Your Complete Exercise Guide*

Breathing Disorders: *Your Complete Exercise Guide*

Chronic Fatigue: *Your Complete Exercise Guide*

Diabetes: *Your Complete Exercise Guide*

Stroke: *Your Complete Exercise Guide*

Chapter 1

What Exercise Can Do for People With Diabetes

It wasn't so long ago when diabetes was spoken about mostly in hushed tones. Pat Gallagher, a Southern California radio-television personality, was first diagnosed with Type I, insulin-dependent diabetes a little over 20 years ago, when he was 14 years old.[1] At the time, Pat was a competitive cross-country runner. However, his doctor shattered Pat's Olympic dreams by erroneously telling him that long-distance running was out of the question for people with diabetes.

Pat felt the weight of his diagnosis so heavily that he didn't admit his disease to anyone—besides family members and his best friend—until 17 years later. Pat is now as forthright as anyone could be about his condition; he hosts a nationally syndicated radio call-in show called "Living with Diabetes," originating from station KFMB in San Diego. Recently, he also began running again and, in fact, has represented the United States in a coast-to-coast relay race across England.

Pat credits his wife, Judy, the radio show's producer, with making him more comfortable with his disease. Judy knew almost nothing about diabetes when she met Pat—but she learned, and she forced him to learn, too. The result of their self-education is this outstanding weekly program, which is now also broadcast on cable television. Among the show's regular features are interviews with celebrities who have diabetes—and there are many. They've ranged from pro golfer Sherri Turner, rock star Bret Michaels, and actor Wilford Brimley to baseball umpire Tom Hallion and quarterback Wade Wilson. And there are many other well-known people with the disease who are scheduled to appear on future shows.

Doing the show has been an eye-opener for Pat. "I had no idea there were so many diabetes-related groups out there—groups for teenagers, for pregnant women, for people on the insulin pump, you name it. Maybe that's the most important function of my show, to let people with diabetes know they're not alone."

CASE HISTORY OF MARK DAVIS

My patient Mark Davis was one of those who became enlightened. Mark was 46 years old, overweight, and out of shape when his doctor told him he had Type II (or non-insulin-dependent) diabetes.

Mark is an investment broker; his white-collar job keeps him planted in a chair for hours at a stretch. A telephone and a computer are the tools of Mark's trade, and, as people familiar with the stock market like to say, his is a job eliciting two intense emotions, fear and greed. Considering his job pressures, Mark seems to be a relatively placid person. But at the time he was diagnosed, he was not a particularly healthy one. His weight had crept up over the years, and he was now almost 45 pounds overweight for his age. He had too high a ratio of body fat to muscle, and the occasional tennis game with his wife or kids had done nothing to maintain his muscle tone.

Mark admitted to his doctor that he hadn't felt his best for years. But what prompted him to schedule an appointment was getting the results of a cholesterol screening test he'd taken one Saturday morning at the local shopping mall. He was shocked to learn that his total cholesterol count was 287 mg/dl, considerably higher than the 200 mg/dl he had been told is the upper limit of the desirable range.* The test renewed a long-standing concern of his wife: Shouldn't you think about losing some weight?

Mark had no obvious symptoms, but he did fit the profile for Type II diabetes: He was middle-aged, he was obese, and he had a family

---

*To convert cholesterol values from milligrams per deciliter (mg/dl) to millimoles per liter (mmol/L), multiply by 0.02586.

history of the disease. When Mark's father was in his late 50s, he developed "a touch of sugar," the misleading euphemism for Type II diabetes. Shortly thereafter, he died of a heart attack—which just goes to show that Type II diabetes can be just as serious as Type I and should never be taken lightly.

Although Mark had no symptoms, his blood and urine tests told the tale. He had glucose in his urine but no ketones. The glucose indicated diabetes, and the lack of ketones suggested that he did not have Type I diabetes. Mark's blood test revealed a high total cholesterol count, with a low concentration of the beneficial high-density lipoprotein (HDL) cholesterol, and elevated levels of triglycerides, another type of fat in the blood. His blood pressure was high (146/95 mmHg) and his fasting blood-glucose count was 237 mg/dl (a normal range is 70 to 114 mg/dl).** It all added up to Type II diabetes.

Mark's doctor explained that diabetes is a chronic disorder of the blood-sugar metabolism that's characterized by excessively high blood-sugar levels. Although there's no cure, Mark could partially reverse his condition if he lost his extra weight through a better diet and exercised regularly. In the short term, such a regimen would enable his body to respond better to the insulin that his pancreas secretes; after all, insulin is the hormone responsible for keeping blood-sugar levels in check. In the long term, it would help Mark avoid the serious complications of diabetes, which include heart and circulatory problems, blindness, and kidney and neurological diseases.

Mark's doctor also told him that with diabetes there are no guarantees. Even if he exercised and ate right, Mark still might need to take special drugs called oral hypoglycemic agents. But even these wouldn't be of optimal benefit if he wasn't also hewing to diet and exercise therapy.

Mark came to the Cooper Clinic determined to change the health habits that contributed to his deteriorating condition. One of our staff dietitians put Mark on a calorie-restricted diet to foster weight loss in tandem with exercise. At first, Mark exercised in a special program supervised by trained medical personnel. By the end of 12 weeks, he was earning the recommended 50 to 100 health points per week. (I'll explain how the Health Points System works in chapter 4.) After that, Mark worked out as a regular member of the Cooper Fitness Center. He was free to do the exercises he enjoyed while also following the guidelines I outline in this book.

**In some countries, blood-glucose values are expressed in millimoles per liter (mmol/L). For glucose values, to convert mg/dl to mmol/L, divide by 18 (for example, 237 mg/dl = 13.2 mmol/L).

Case history, Mark Davis

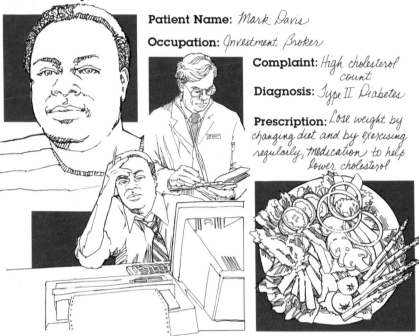

Patient Name: *Mark Davis*

Occupation: *Investment Broker*

Complaint: *High cholesterol count*

Diagnosis: *Type II Diabetes*

Prescription: *Lose weight by changing diet and by exercising regularly, medication to help lower cholesterol*

After 6 months, Mark was exercising 5 days a week, doing mostly brisk walking and riding on a stationary cycle that worked both his arms and legs. His steady efforts to earn 50 to 100 health points weekly were already paying dividends. He'd lost over 20 pounds and was determined to continue losing about 1 pound a week. His blood pressure was normal, and his fasting blood-glucose level was around 130 mg/dl, close to normal. His physician told him that if he kept up the good work, there was a good chance he'd never have to take drugs to lower his blood sugar, as many people with Type II diabetes do.

But Mark's doctor did prescribe a drug for Mark's cholesterol problem. Many diabetes patients develop heart disease, and Mark's father had died from it. Exercise and diet had helped Mark's blood-lipid levels, to be sure: His total cholesterol had decreased by 15% to 244 mg/dl, his triglycerides were down 30%, and his good HDL cholesterol had gone up by almost 10%. But these numbers still weren't good enough.

Today, Mark looks and feels better than he has in years. And he says his diligence has delivered a nice bonus: He is more productive at work and enjoys life more.

CASE HISTORY OF LINDA STONE

I first heard about Linda from her uncle, Mike Stone, a patient in our cardiac rehabilitation program. One morning some months after his heart attack, Mike told me about Linda as he pedaled away on a stationary cycle. He said that at a family gathering over the weekend everyone had commented on how good he looked. He'd credited the transformation to his new habit of regular exercise. Linda had listened, then expressed doubts the exercise prescription could work for her because of her "special circumstances."

Linda's special circumstances were Type I diabetes. Since the age of 16, she'd been on daily insulin injections. Her very life depended on her ability to keep her blood-sugar levels from rising too high (a condition known as *hyperglycemia*) or falling too low (*hypoglycemia*), either of which could be fatal. Exercise made this balancing act all the more difficult. And her physician had told her that although exercise could help a person with Type II diabetes to achieve better blood-glucose control (by making the body more sensitive to the insulin that the pancreas produces), the same could not be said for a person with Type I diabetes whose pancreas no longer secretes any insulin whatsoever.

Mike, an exercise enthusiast, wanted to know if all this was true. I explained to Mike that because modern technology enables people to easily monitor their own blood-sugar levels, most people with Type I diabetes—such as Linda—can exercise safely. Linda's doctor is right that exercise makes optimal blood-glucose control a challenge for people with Type I diabetes, but that doesn't mean exercise is out of the question. Type I diabetes patients simply need to work with their health-care team to adjust their insulin dosages appropriately. (Health-care teams—comprised of a medical doctor/specialist, nurse educator, dietitian, and other health professionals—are the most common mode of diabetes management today. With their help, amazing things are possible.)

Because heart disease runs in the Stone family, I also told Mike that it was especially important for Linda to start exercising; otherwise she'd be more likely to have a heart attack at a rather young age, as Mike did.

Linda listened to her uncle and came in to see me. Her history was rather typical for a person with Type I diabetes. For the first 10 years after her diagnosis, she was on conventional insulin therapy, following a split-mixed regimen: She injected mixtures of regular, short-acting insulin and intermediate-acting insulin before breakfast and dinner each day. Just before the birth of her daughter 4 years earlier, she'd switched to intensive insulin therapy, which mainly involves self-monitoring blood-sugar levels and injecting appropriate amounts of regular insulin before each meal. Based on trial and error and in consultation with her health-care team, Linda had learned how to adjust the insulin dosages to her diet and anticipated physical activity.

Linda was quite competent at self-monitoring, so she was an ideal candidate for a regular exercise program. But I eased her into it slowly until she learned exactly how her body responded. She welcomed our help because she'd already tried aerobic dance on her own with somewhat disastrous results. On three occasions she'd had hypo-glycemic reactions several hours after a particularly strenuous class. The third occasion was the last time she'd bothered with any form of exercise in more than 2 years.

As Mark did, Linda started in our 12-week supervised exercise program. Our medical staff worked closely with her on food intake and adjustments to her insulin dosages to insure there would be no more hypoglycemia surprises. By the end of the program, Linda knew

---

Case history, Linda Stone

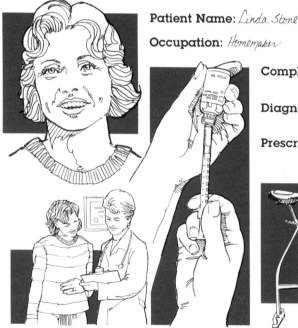

Patient Name: *Linda Stone*

Occupation: *Homemaker*

Complaint: *Lack of energy*

Diagnosis: *Type I Diabetes*

Prescription:
Exercise

how her body reacted to when and what she ate in relation to her exertion.

Linda graduated to exercise self-reliance and our Health Points System. Today, a year after she first came to me, Linda has been exercising regularly and vigorously; she has yet to have a serious hypoglycemic reaction. Yes, she's had a few mild reactions, but she knows what to do to halt them and get her blood sugar immediately back up to manageable levels. Linda reports that she now feels better, has more energy, sleeps more soundly, and has an improved self-image. She is no longer anxious or depressed about her condition. And she feels more at ease, knowing that she's doing something constructive to reduce her risk of developing diabetes complications.

From a physiological perspective, these improvements are understandable. Because regular exercise has made the cells in Linda's body more sensitive to the insulin she injects, she's been able to cut the dosage by more than 10%, and her blood-glucose control is as good as it ever was. Her fitness level, which is measured at the Cooper Clinic via treadmill exercise testing, has increased by more than 25% since she began our program.

For a person with Type I diabetes, the purpose of exercise is not so much to control blood-sugar levels as to stave off long-term complications and improve general fitness and outlook on life. These same reasons motivate most people who exercise, whether or not they have diabetes.

DIABETES IN PROFILE

In introducing you to Mark and Linda, I have discussed two types of diabetes; there are actually three.

Insulin-dependent diabetes mellitus is also referred to as Type I or IDDM. Another name, *juvenile-onset diabetes*, isn't used anymore because it gives a false impression. Although people are generally under 30 years old when they're diagnosed, Type I diabetes can develop at any age. In this disorder, the body is either completely unable to produce insulin, which controls blood-glucose levels, or able to produce such a tiny amount that insulin injections are still necessary. About 1 million people in the United States have Type I diabetes.

Non-insulin-dependent diabetes mellitus (Type II or NIDDM) was previously referred to as *adult-onset diabetes* for good reason: People generally (but not always) are older than 30 when they learn they have it. Type II diabetes is widespread; up to 10 million people in the United States have it.

In Type II diabetes, the pancreas still secretes insulin; indeed, insulin levels in the blood may be normal or even excessive. But the body doesn't respond properly to insulin's action, an abnormality that's often termed *insulin resistance* or *reduced insulin sensitivity*. In extreme cases, people with Type II diabetes need to supplement their natural insulin production with insulin injections. But that is the exception, not the rule. It's much more common for a person with Type II diabetes to be on oral hypoglycemic agents, drugs that are not insulin but still help to keep blood-glucose levels within a normal range.

The third type of diabetes is the rarest. It has no special name because it's actually a variety of other medical conditions or diseases (among them, chronic pancreatitis, cystic fibrosis, Cushing's syndrome, and hemochromatosis) that can result in impaired insulin secretion or action, or both. Patients on certain medications, such as some blood-pressure-lowering drugs, may also fall into this category.

There are occasional exceptions to what I've just outlined. Nearly all patients who are under the age of 20 at the time of diagnosis have Type I diabetes, but this type can develop at any age—and does. Similarly, I've known cases where a child or adolescent develops Type II diabetes (which goes by the somewhat awkward name of *maturity-onset diabetes of the young*, or MODY). However, these exceptions are uncommon.

AN OVERVIEW OF DIABETES TREATMENT AND REHABILITATION

Whether you have Type I or Type II diabetes, I believe the best approach to managing it is to work toward these three goals:

- To return your blood-sugar metabolism to optimal levels as soon as possible—and then to make sure the levels fluctuate daily within a narrow range that mimics that of healthy people. Once you accomplish this, you'll be less likely to have a blood-sugar emergency.
- To take the precautions that can help prevent complications, many of which are as serious—and potentially fatal—as diabetes itself. For example, be vigilant about stabilizing your blood pressure, cholesterol levels, and weight. Also, exercise regularly, stop smoking (if you smoke), and take special care of your feet.

- To develop a healthy lifestyle and outlook that's not limited by diabetes strictures and dictates—or as Pat Gallagher says, "To control your diabetes instead of letting it control you."

My goal in writing this book is to help you help yourself accomplish these three objectives. It may not be easy at first. After all, an uncomfortable learning curve accompanies most things in life that are worthwhile but challenging. However, I believe that almost anyone who is properly motivated can be vital despite diabetes.

You might want to think of this slim volume as your diabetes exercise guidebook. As you'll discover, I'm not advocating rules for their own sake. Yes, I want you to know as much as possible about your condition and what exercise can do to alleviate it. But I also want you to take control of your situation and find ways to shape my exercise guidelines to your lifestyle. Ideally, I want you to follow the pattern of the typical diabetes patient who is a member of The Cooper Aerobics Center: They work out faithfully, watch what they eat, and take their prescribed medications. They're active, involved people—who just happen to have diabetes.

Chapter 2

Exercise Benefits for People With Diabetes

The notion of exercise as a form of diabetes treatment and rehabilitation is hardly a new one. The Indian physician Sushruta advocated it as early as 600 B.C.[1] In the ensuing centuries, the pendulum has swung back and forth several times—treatment for diabetes has wavered between exercise as therapy and the exact opposite, complete bed rest. Today, researchers know that the notion of bed rest as diabetes therapy is a fallacy. Studies have shown that lying in bed for even 7 days impairs the body's blood-sugar metabolism.

In the early 1900s, diabetes researchers finally found the hard evidence they needed to justify the use of exercise for diabetes rehabilitation. In 1919 (after the measurement of blood-glucose levels became routine), researchers proved that a short bout of exercise could depress blood-glucose levels.[2] Insulin medication was developed in 1921. Soon thereafter, in a 1926 article in the *British Medical Journal*, R.D. Lawrence reported that exercise could enhance the blood-glucose-lowering effects of injected insulin, thus decreasing the insulin needs of Type I diabetes patients.[3] It was Lawrence's study results, which doctors of the time saw borne out in their own exercising patients' experiences, that ignited strong contemporary interest in regular exercise as a cornerstone of diabetes treatment.

Over the last two decades, investigators have continued to do extensive exercise-diabetes research. Consequently, doctors have retreated somewhat from the position that all diabetes patients are candidates for the exercise prescription. Strenuous workouts are definitely risky for some people, depending on their diabetes complications. And those with Type I diabetes should not be led to believe that exercise will consistently improve their blood-sugar control. It might not.

These caveats do not mean I'm turning a thumbs-down on exercise for a broad group of diabetes patients. But people with diabetes who exercise must understand how exertion affects blood-glucose metabolism so they'll know how it will affect them. They should also know what they can do to gain the most benefits from regular exercise while minimizing the risks. Keep in mind that exercise carries a small risk of injury for everyone, not just for people with diabetes.

Your diabetes exercise program should address these goals:

- To help you control your blood sugar
- To maintain your ideal weight
- To improve your quality of life
- To avoid developing diabetes complications

REGULATES BLOOD SUGAR

Recent studies of people who don't have diabetes have shown that insulin sensitivity—the cell's ability to respond to insulin and to take up sugar from the blood—is greater in physically fit people than in those who are unfit. And regular exercise can help reverse the usual decline in insulin sensitivity that occurs with aging.

How Exercise Affects Type I Diabetes Patients' Blood-Sugar Control

The same applies to a person with Type I diabetes who is on conventional or intensive insulin therapy. Exercise can increase that person's insulin sensitivity, which can be very beneficial.[4] But better cellular sensitivity does not automatically mean better blood-sugar control. In separate studies in Toronto, Canada, and Stockholm, Sweden, 12 to

16 weeks of exercise training failed to improve fasting blood-glucose and glycosylated-hemoglobin levels* in Type I diabetes patients.[5,6] However, the study methods used may have influenced the results. On exercise days, if subjects didn't eat more before their workouts as a preventive strategy against hypoglycemia, some of them certainly ate excessive amounts afterward.

The results were quite different in an 8-week study by Ron Stratton and his colleagues at the H. Allen Chapman Research Institute of Medical Genetics in Tulsa, OK.[7] They studied 8 adolescents with Type I diabetes. The subjects worked out for 30 to 45 minutes 5 days a week. Exercise was scheduled after the regular afternoon snack and before the evening meal, and subjects were discouraged from eating extra food before exercise. Rather than having the subjects routinely eat extra food before exercise sessions, the investigators reduced subjects' insulin dosages before workouts and let them eat additional food afterward, but only when it was necessary to prevent hypoglycemia. By the last 3 weeks of the study, the teenagers' blood-glucose levels before the exercise sessions were significantly lower than their levels during the first 3 weeks (161 mg/dl vs. 198 mg/dl). In 5 of the 8 study participants, daily insulin dosages were reduced across the board, not just on exercise days. The subjects' glycosylated-hemoglobin values did not improve, perhaps because of the truncated study period, but their levels of *glycosylated serum albumin*, a more sensitive index of blood-glucose changes over a shorter interval, showed a marked decline.

On the basis of such studies, I believe regular exercise can help improve blood-sugar control somewhat, provided that Type I diabetes patients don't change their diet on workout days unless it's really necessary and that they pay attention to other important factors, such as (a) the time of day when exercise is performed; (b) the duration and intensity of the exercise; (c) the precise blood-glucose level immediately prior to exercise; (d) fitness level, irrespective of the diabetes; and (e) the type and dosage of the insulin injected. To truly get the optimum

---

*For a truly accurate assessment of blood-glucose control, one of the best methods is a glycosylated-hemoglobin test. When glucose in the blood attaches to hemoglobin, contained in red blood cells, it forms glycosylated hemoglobin. The higher your blood-glucose level, the more glycosylated hemoglobin there will be in your blood. Red blood cells usually live for about 120 days (4 months); the average age of those circulating in your bloodstream is 2 months. Therefore, the concentration of glycosylated hemoglobin in the blood at any given time is considered a good measure of a person's average blood glucose level over the preceding 6 to 10 weeks. This is why this test is often called "the blood test with a memory."

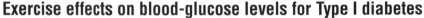

Exercise effects on blood-glucose levels for Type I diabetes

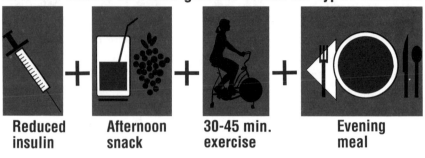

| Reduced insulin | Afternoon snack | 30-45 min. exercise | Evening meal |

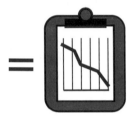

Lower blood-glucose levels after 5 weeks

diabetes-management benefits from exercise over the long term, a person with Type I diabetes would have to train every day, preferably after a meal, at a set intensity and duration. Doing this would restrict that person's lifestyle even more than it is already. So I agree with those who no longer consider exercise to be the primary means for achieving optimal blood-glucose control in people with Type I diabetes —especially when it can be achieved by the far simpler method of altering insulin dosages based on self-monitoring results. But, for reasons I will soon outline, I do still consider regular exercise to be extremely valuable for people with Type I diabetes.

How Exercise Affects Type II Diabetes Patients' Blood-Sugar Control

The reservations I expressed about the advantages of exercise for Type I diabetes patients do not hold for those with Type II diabetes. Quite the contrary. For those with Type II, exercise should be a primary means of blood-glucose control. On the priority list, it comes right after eating correctly. Studies show conclusively that a regular exercise program is of great value in controlling blood-sugar levels in people with Type II diabetes.

Recently, epidemiological studies (which look at the occurrence of disease in large populations) have revealed alarmingly high rates of Type II diabetes—more than 20% of all adults—in parts of the world where this condition was once rare. Heredity alone cannot account for such high prevalence rates. Affected populations include the Pima Indians and other North American Indians, Tamil-speaking East Indians in South Africa, and some Micronesians and Melanesians from the Pacific region.

What do they have in common? They tend to eat too much and exercise too little.[8]

Epidemiological studies have also shown that increased physical activity is effective in preventing Type II diabetes. And the protective benefit of regular exercise seems to be especially pronounced in those at the highest risk for the disease: persons who are obese, persons with high blood pressure, and children of persons with diabetes.[9]

The results of exercise studies of Type II diabetes subjects are unequivocal: Regular exercise can improve blood-glucose control and glycosylated-hemoglobin levels. Perhaps the most telling study is a 10-year one that compared blood-glucose levels in 100 Type II diabetes patients, about half of whom exercised regularly and the remainder of whom did not. At the completion, researchers documented much lower blood-sugar and glycosylated-hemoglobin values in the exercisers.[10]

The results of the 10-year study aren't that surprising because exercise is known to improve insulin sensitivity. One reason people develop Type II diabetes in the first place is that their cells have grown resistant, or insensitive, to the insulin in their blood. Insulin resistance, rather than a complete lack of insulin, is a major cause of elevated blood-sugar levels in Type II diabetes patients.

But exercise alone is not the answer. Another study, conducted by Clifton Bogardus and colleagues at the University of Vermont, showed that the right diet combined with regular exercise is the best method for improving blood-glucose control in Type II diabetes patients. These researchers found that different and better metabolic pathways to blood-glucose control are triggered when both approaches are employed in tandem.[11]

HELPS MAINTAIN IDEAL WEIGHT

Shedding pounds is no easy task, but it's essential for any diabetes patient who is overweight. It's so important that a 1987 report from a

National Institutes of Health consensus development panel pinpointed weight reduction as the key nutritional goal for any overweight person with Type II diabetes.[12] Weight loss improves blood-glucose control by lowering the liver's glucose production and increasing insulin sensitivity. It can also boost pancreatic insulin secretions. *Reducing weight to within the ideal range is often the only treatment that Type II diabetes patients need to normalize their blood-glucose levels.*

If you weigh too much, one of the principal reasons to exercise faithfully is to bring your weight down into the ideal range and, once you get it there, to help keep it there. Exercise is critical to the success of a weight-loss program for several reasons.

As you know, we burn calories more quickly when we exercise than when we are sedentary. Regular exercise is also thought to help keep our *resting metabolic rate* (RMR) operating at a lively clip, and that's especially important when you're on a calorie-restricted diet. When you eat fewer calories and don't exercise, your RMR slows in response to what your body interprets as starvation conditions. This slower RMR accounts for the plateau effect many crash dieters experience within a few weeks of starting a diet. Their metabolism winds down

How weight loss improves blood-glucose control

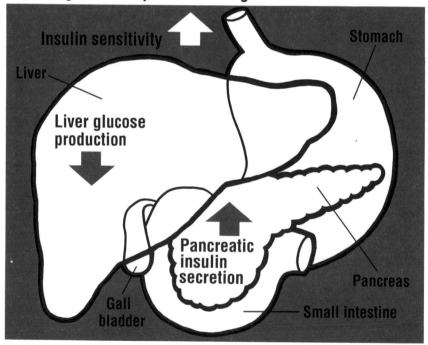

to adjust to the meager food rations and to conserve the body's fat-fuel stores as long as possible. If your goal is weight loss, this is precisely what you do *not* want your body to do.

Exercise also helps ensure that we retain our good lean-body mass. Studies show that as much as 25% of weight lost through dieting alone is lean-body mass.[13] That means an undesirable loss of vital tissues—muscle, bone, and other metabolically active tissue. It's dead-weight body fat you want to shed, not protein tissue.

Finally, exercise is the key to maintaining your ideal weight in the long term. A Stanford University School of Medicine study found that it's easier to maintain weight lost through exercise than it is to maintain weight lost through diet alone.[14] Nonetheless, I think the best approach is a combination of the two.

IMPROVES QUALITY OF LIFE

There's no question that exercise helps most people with diabetes improve their psychological well-being. How exercise fits into a diabetes patient's life was summarized best in the September/October 1988 edition of *Diabetes Spectrum*. The commentary concluded by stating that to say that exercise isn't of much value to people with diabetes because it doesn't carry an ironclad guarantee to aid in blood-glucose control is "like not seeing the forest for the trees." When you place exercise within the big picture of your lifestyle, its value goes way beyond the issue of blood-sugar levels.[15]

Diabetes can affect you psychologically as well as physically. Some of the complications of diabetes, such as premature disability or sudden death, can be pretty stressful just to think about. And diabetes treatment makes unrelenting demands which, in severe cases, can disrupt the ordinary functioning of a person's life.

Exercise can help ease the strains and tension you may feel, both because of your illness and just because everyday life is stressful. Most health professionals, including me, have witnessed the change in outlook in diabetes patients who take on a regular exercise program. They feel better, sleep better, have more energy, and feel more self-confident. Staying on a program also convinces them they have good self-discipline and self-control, important traits for people who must adhere strictly to a diabetes management regimen. For children and adolescents with diabetes, participation in sports not only confers the benefits I just mentioned, but it also gives them a marvelous sense of accomplishment and a way to meet new friends.

In adults, regular exercise also goes a long way toward relieving anxiety and depression—which is why Ken Cooper touts it as "nature's own tranquilizer."

HELPS PREVENT THE DEVELOPMENT OF DIABETES COMPLICATIONS

From a purely physiological standpoint, exercise can have a profoundly positive impact on your body. It can also have a negative impact and worsen or bring on some of the chronic complications of diabetes, if adequate precautions aren't taken. Table 2.1 provides a short glossary to the most common, potentially life-threatening cardiac, vascular, and neurological complications.

After reading through the list of complications, you may feel the need for a stiff drink—which may be unwise if you've got diabetes. There's cause for cheer of a nonliquid source, however. Today, there is strong evidence that good diabetes control can help you prevent the onset of complications.[16] There are people alive today who have had diabetes for more than 50 years and have never developed any serious complications. Such cases are becoming more and more common.

Exercise done properly can be of enormous value in preventing or alleviating many of these complications. This fact is supported by preliminary findings from a major research study in progress at The Cooper Institute for Aerobics Research (see Figure 2.1).

Of the various diabetes complications, coronary artery disease causes the most deaths in persons with diabetes. In 1987, Kenneth E. Powell and his colleagues at the Centers for Disease Control scrutinized more than 40 respected studies, dating back to 1950, on physical activity and coronary artery disease prevention. Their goal was to assess how, and if, exercise can prevent deaths from heart disease.[17] They concluded that physical inactivity is as strong a risk factor for premature death from heart disease as the traditional risk factors you hear so much about—cigarette smoking, high blood pressure, and high cholesterol.

Several studies completed since the publication of Powell's overview strongly support the Powell group's conclusion. The evidence is compelling that regular exercise can reduce the risk of dying from heart disease by almost 50%.[18] For this reason, the American Heart Association now considers physical inactivity, or lack of regular exercise, to

Table 2.1
Glossary of Diabetes Complications

Complication	Brief description
Coronary artery disease	This condition, caused by atherosclerotic plaque buildup in the coronary arteries, results in too little blood and oxygen reaching the heart muscle. Sometimes it's accompanied by symptoms such as chest pain or discomfort. Other times, it's asymptomatic, or silent. Left untreated, coronary artery disease can result in a heart attack or even sudden death.
Intermittent claudication	This complication is caused by the buildup of atherosclerotic plaque in the arteries to the legs, a condition called *peripheral vascular disease*. The symptoms are pain or lameness (*claudication*) in the buttocks or legs, which is only felt during exercise. It's relieved by rest, which is why it's termed *intermittent*.
Diabetic retinopathy	This is a progressive disease (*pathy*) that damages the retina (*retino*). The retina is the area inside the eye that acts like a camera and records images of objects to relay to the brain. The first two stages of the disease—*background* and *preproliferative* retinopathy—often have no symptoms, although during these stages the retinal blood vessels are slowly becoming nonfunctional. Left untreated, the condition becomes *proliferative* as new blood vessels form in an attempt to maintain an adequate blood supply to the retina. Because they're very fragile, the blood vessels rupture easily, reducing vision and finally causing blindness.
Diabetic nephropathy	This disease of the kidneys (*nephro*) is caused by damage to the kidneys' small blood vessels. The visible signs are excretion of protein in the urine, swelling of the feet and ankles, and high blood pressure. Left unchecked, this condition results in kidney failure.
Peripheral neuropathy	Disease of the nerves that control sensation and, to a lesser degree, the nerves that control muscle functioning.
Autonomic neuropathy	Disease affecting the *autonomic* nerves, the nerves that we don't consciously control. The autonomic nerves of the body are important because they exert influence over key internal organs, such as the heart.

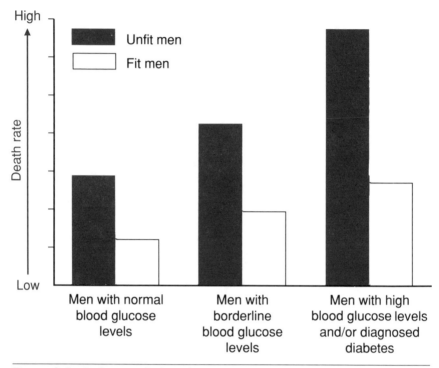

Figure 2.1   Preliminary findings from a major research study involving 8,118 male Cooper Clinic patients. The study compared death rates among physically fit and unfit men during an average follow-up of 8 years. Comparisons are shown for men with normal blood-glucose levels, borderline blood-glucose levels, and high blood-glucose levels or diagnosed diabetes. In each group, death rates were lower for the fit than the unfit men. For the men with high blood-glucose levels or diagnosed diabetes, death rates were more than 2.5 times greater in the unfit than the fit men. Also note that the death rate for the fit men with high blood-glucose levels or diagnosed diabetes is no higher than that for the unfit men with normal blood-glucose levels.

be the fourth major risk factor for coronary artery disease (the other three are cigarette smoking, high blood pressure, and high cholesterol).[19]

The box that follows outlines the pros and cons of exercise for all people with diabetes, no matter which type. In the chapters that follow, I will show you how to minimize your risks and optimize your benefits. Keep in mind that exercise is a double-edged sword. Use it wisely, for good rather than ill.

THE PLUSES AND MINUSES OF EXERCISE
FOR ALL PEOPLE WITH DIABETES

You can derive these 13 crucial, health-promoting benefits from regular exercise:

+ Improved insulin sensitivity
+ Better functional capacity, the ability to perform everyday tasks with ease
+ Enhanced sense of well-being
+ Less risk of developing coronary artery disease
+ Reduced risk of death from a heart attack
+ Lowered need of the heart for oxygen during exercise
+ Lessened stickiness of blood platelets, thus less chance of blood-clot formation
+ Lowered long-term risk of developing high blood pressure and a lowering of blood-pressure levels that are already elevated
+ Reduced triglyceride levels
+ Rise in high-density lipoprotein cholesterol, the good HDL cholesterol
+ Healthier total cholesterol to HDL-cholesterol ratio
+ Reduction in body fat, hence reduced obesity
+ Reduced risk of developing osteoporosis

Exercise, however, is not risk-free. Diabetes patients face these potential risks:

− Hypoglycemia, for people taking insulin or oral hypoglycemic agents
− Hyperglycemia and, for those with Type I, ketoacidosis
− Cardiac complications, including sudden death
− Retinal bleeding in the eye
− Protein excreted in the urine
− Excessive vacillation, up or down, in the systolic blood pressure
− Greater risk of developing foot ulcers and orthopedic injuries, especially in people with peripheral neuropathy
− Steep rise in body temperature

Chapter 2
Prescription

❐ Include exercise in your diabetes treatment and rehabilitation program.

❐ Exercise regularly to reduce your risk for long-term diabetes complications and premature death.

❐ Exercise regularly to help improve your blood-sugar control.

❐ Exercise regularly to help reach and maintain your ideal body weight.

❐ Exercise regularly to improve your quality of life.

❐ Keep in mind that exercise is not a panacea but an extremely important supplemental therapy.

❐ To gain optimal benefits, combine regular exercise with appropriate medical care and other positive lifestyle changes.

❐ Be aware that inappropriate exercise could worsen your diabetes and any complications stemming from it.

❐ Obtain your doctor's consent before beginning an exercise program.

Chapter 3

Getting Started on a Regular Exercise Program

You might want to think of exercise as a form of diabetes medication. When you exercise, just as when you take a drug, you must strike a fine balance between two goals: effectiveness and safety. In this chapter and the next, I'll focus on effectiveness. I'll explain which types of exercise and how much of each you need to do for maximum health benefits. In chapters 5 and 6, I'll go on to discuss safety.

COMPONENTS OF AN EXERCISE WORKOUT

A typical exercise session should consist of the following parts: 10 to 20 minutes of stretching and muscle strengthening, 5 minutes of aerobic warm-up, 15 to 60 minutes of aerobic exercise at an appropriate intensity, 5 minutes of aerobic cool-down, and, finally, 5 minutes of stretching. Note that stretching and muscle strengthening are included at the beginning, and stretching exercises are repeated at the end of the workout. Please keep in mind that it may take you several weeks to work your way up to the durations I've specified.

What's the reason for doing all these forms of exercise? The aerobic portion of the workout, of course, is aimed squarely at reducing your risk for chronic diabetes complications and increasing your body's sensitivity to insulin. Yes, it's the most important. But stretching and strengthening your muscles shouldn't be overlooked, either. After all, without well-functioning muscles, you can't do aerobics—or many other recreational, occupational, and self-care activities. Also, without strong, flexible muscles, you're more likely to incur a musculoskeletal injury. And by increasing your muscle mass, strengthening exercises may increase your insulin sensitivity.[1] (For more information on the benefits of muscle strengthening, see *The Strength Connection*, a recent book by The Cooper Institute for Aerobics Research.[2])

Stretching Exercises

Stretching is part of a good exercise protocol. It should always precede an aerobic exercise session, whether you have diabetes or not. It won't take you long to appreciate the value of stretching. It relaxes you mentally and physically and probably helps prevent injuries by increasing your flexibility and widening your freedom of movement.

At the beginning of an exercise session, and if you have time at the end (and I encourage you to make time), do the stretches shown and described in Figures 3.1-3.5. Each stretch should be held for 10 to 20 seconds with no bouncing. Do not stretch to the point where the exercise becomes painful. Remember to keep breathing regularly—do not hold your breath. Over the years, I have found these exercises to be particularly useful. But if you have any musculoskeletal problems, such as arthritis, please check with your doctor before doing them.

Shoulder and Back Stretch.   Lift your right elbow toward the ceiling and place your right hand as far down your back between the shoulder blades as possible. Allow your chin to rest on your chest. If possible, using your left hand, gently pull your right elbow to the left until a stretch is felt on the back of the right arm and down the right side of the back. Hold. Repeat with the left arm.

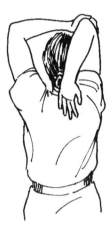

Figure 3.1

Inner Thigh Stretch.   Sit on the floor, place the soles of your feet together, and pull your heels in as close to the buttocks as possible. Gently press your knees down toward the floor.

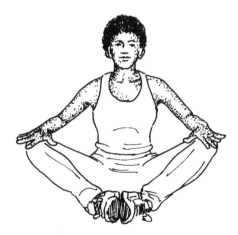

Figure 3.2

Lower Back and Hamstring Stretch.   Sitting on the floor with your legs straight out in front of you and your hands on your thighs, bend forward slowly, reaching toward your toes. Keep your head and back aligned as you move into the stretch. If necessary, you can bend your knees slightly.

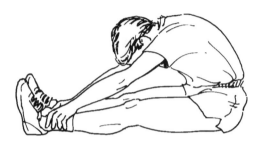

Figure 3.3

Lower Back, Thigh, and Hip Stretch.   Lie flat on your back with your legs extended on the floor. Pull your right knee up to your chest and press your back to the floor. Hold this position and then repeat with the left knee.

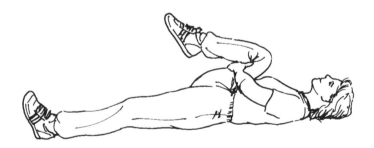

Figure 3.4

Calf Stretch. Stand facing a wall, approximately three feet away. Place your palms on the wall, keeping your feet flat on the floor. Leave one foot in place as you step forward with the other. Make sure your back remains straight as you gently bend the front knee forward toward the wall. Repeat the same exercise with the opposite leg.

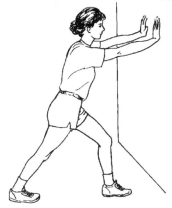

Figure 3.5

Muscle-Strengthening Exercises

In contrast to flexibility training, which you should include in all your workouts, muscle-strengthening exercises need to be done only 2 or 3 days a week—and *not* on consecutive days. Even this minimal amount of strength training may be too much for some diabetes patients, though. Although it's safe for people with uncomplicated diabetes, muscle strengthening with heavy weights can cause an excessive rise in blood pressure that can be dangerous for anyone with cardiac, vascular, or neurological complications. If you fall into this category yet you've received clearance from your doctor to proceed with muscle strengthening, pay special attention to the following words of caution:

• *Don't hold a contraction for more than about 6 seconds.* Isometric exercise—a static type of muscle-strengthening exercise in which a muscle remains contracted for more than a few seconds without relaxing—can elicit adverse cardiac responses in patients with cardiac, vascular, or neurological complications.

• *Avoid holding your breath.* A Valsalva maneuver during lifting—that is, exhaling forcefully without releasing the air from the lungs—is ill-advised because it places increased stress on your cardiovascular system.

• *Do not undertake activities where you must hold weight above your head for more than a few seconds.* Such movements also place an excessive load on your cardiovascular system.

• *Substitute lighter weights for heavier weights and do more repetitions.* Do not use heavier weights with the idea that you'll just exercise for a shorter time. Heavier weights increase your blood pressure to a greater degree than lighter ones.

I've developed an easy muscle-strengthening program that most people with diabetes can do at home with minimal risk. It's based on the use of light hand-held weights, ranging from a beginning weight of 1.5 to 6 pounds (about 0.5 to 3 kilograms) to a top weight of 13 pounds (about 6 kilograms). The program works all the major muscles and takes the previously mentioned cautions into account. Although this program was designed for patients with cardiac, vascular, and neurological complications, you should still check with your doctor before starting it. The program is shown in Figures 3.6-3.16. (Incidentally, it's fine if you do muscle strengthening after, rather than before, the aerobic portion of your workout.)

I recommend that you perform these exercises 3 days a week on alternate days and follow these guidelines:

- Begin with a hand-held weight no heavier than 6 pounds (about 3 kilograms), and gradually progress to a maximum weight of 13 pounds (about 6 kilograms) if you can.
- Do 8 to 16 complete and continuous executions, or repetitions, for each exercise.
- Perform each exercise one or two times and rest 15 to 60 seconds between sets. Once you've reached the point where you can perform two complete sets (2×16 repetitions for each exercise) with relative ease, you may want to try a heavier weight. But it's more important to do the exercise correctly than to increase the amount of weight.
- Do not hold your breath during these repetitions. If you feel inclined to do so, the weight may be too heavy. You may be straining too much.
- Maintain good posture throughout each exercise set.

Side Shoulder Raise (outer portion of the shoulder).   Start with your arms hanging in front of your thighs, elbows slightly bent, and palms facing each other. Raise both dumbbells outwards simultaneously to shoulder height, keeping elbows slightly bent. Lower dumbbells to starting position and repeat.

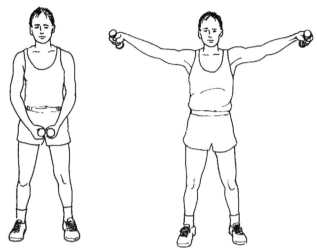

Figure 3.6

Front Shoulder Raise (front portion of the shoulder).   Begin with your arms hanging in front of your thighs and your palms facing the thighs. Raise one dumbbell straight in front of you to shoulder height. Lower this dumbbell to your starting position and repeat using your other arm. Keep alternating your arms.

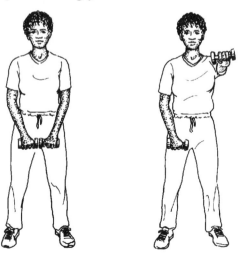

Figure 3.7

Bent-Over Shoulder Raise (rear portion of the shoulder and upper back).   Bend over until your torso is roughly parallel to floor. Keep your knees slightly bent. Start with your arms hanging down towards the floor, palms facing inward, and elbows slightly bent. Raise both dumbbells outwards simultaneously to shoulder height, keeping your elbows slightly bent. Lower the dumbbells to starting position and repeat.

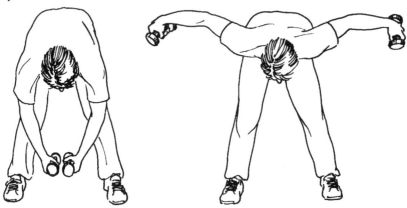

Figure 3.8

Upright Row (shoulder, neck, and upper back).   Stand with your arms hanging in front of your thighs, palms facing your thighs, and the dumbbells close together. Keeping your palms close to the body, raise the dumbbells simultaneously to your chin. Lower the dumbbells to starting position and repeat.

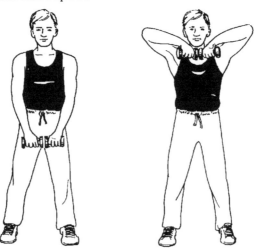

Figure 3.9

Biceps Curl (biceps, or front of upper arm). Start the exercise with your arms hanging at your sides and your palms facing in front of you. Keeping the elbows close to the sides of the body, curl both dumbbells upward to the shoulders. Lower and repeat.

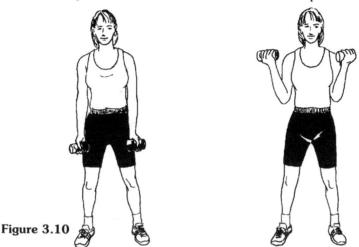

Figure 3.10

Triceps Extension (triceps, or back of upper arm). Place one foot about a step in front of the other and bend both knees slightly. Lean forward and rest one hand, palm down, on the knee of your front leg. Place the hand with the dumbbell in it against your hip (palm of your hand facing the hip). Keeping your elbow still, straighten your arm fully. Then bend your arm until it returns to your hip and repeat. After completing the desired number of repetitions, repeat with the other arm.

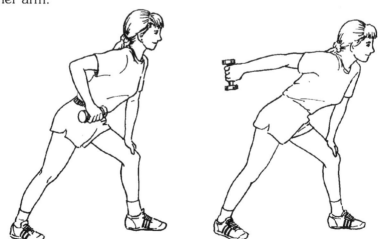

Figure 3.11

Supine Fly (chest muscles). Lie face up on the floor. Place your arms perpendicular to your body. Raise both dumbbells up above your chest to meet in the center. Lower the dumbbells and repeat.

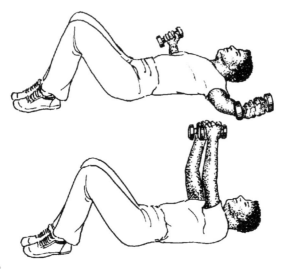

Figure 3.12

Pullover (chest and back). Lie face up on the floor. Begin with the dumbbells held together directly above the center of your chest, with your elbows slightly bent. Lower the dumbbells to the floor behind your head, keeping your elbows bent. Raise the dumbbells back to starting position and repeat.

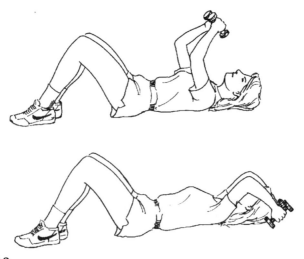

Figure 3.13

Sit Ups (abdominal muscles). From a horizontal position with your knees bent at a 90-degree angle and the palms of your hands resting on your thighs, lift your shoulders off the ground and slide your fingers up toward your knees. Return to starting position and repeat.

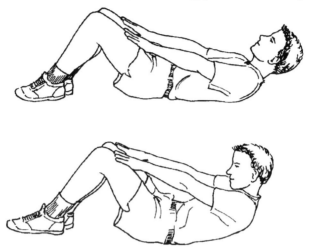

Figure 3.14

Calf Raises (calf muscles). Start with your arms hanging at your sides, dumbbells in hand, and feet only slightly apart. Raise up onto the balls of both feet. Lower your heels to the ground and repeat. Do not bend your knees.

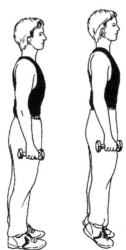

Figure 3.15

Lunges (thigh muscles and buttocks).   Start with your arms hanging at your sides, dumbbells in hands, and feet apart. Take one step forward with one foot and bend your front knee slightly. Step back to starting position and repeat with the opposite leg.

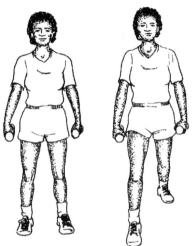

Figure 3.16

If your doctor clears you for a more strenuous muscle-strengthening program, find a health professional who is familiar with your case and adequately trained to instruct you in the correct use of resistance-training equipment. A well-equipped gym might be outfitted with weight-training devices carrying such brand names as Cybex Strength Systems, Hydrafitness, Nautilus, and Universal. These are excellent machines, but someone should carefully instruct you how to use them and supervise your exercise.

The American College of Sports Medicine recommends that the average adult perform a minimum of 8 to 10 exercises using the major muscle groups at least twice weekly.[3] The college further encourages adults to perform at least one set, consisting of 8 to 12 repetitions, of each exercise in a muscle-strengthening workout. These recommendations are appropriate for people with diabetes. But if you have both diabetes and heart disease, I suggest you consult *The Cooper Clinic Cardiac Rehabilitation Program* for more extensive guidelines.[4]

Aerobic Exercise

Ken Cooper coined the term *aerobics* in 1968 when his first book, *Aerobics*, was published.[5] If you'd looked up the word *aerobic* in the dictionary before 1968, it would have been described as an adjective meaning "growing in air or oxygen." It was commonly used to describe bacteria that need oxygen to live. Ken, however, used the word *aerobics* as a noun to denote those forms of endurance exercises that require increased amounts of oxygen for prolonged periods of time. Proof of Ken's influence came in the 1986 edition of the *Oxford English Dictionary*, which defines *aerobics* as "a method of physical exercise for producing beneficial changes in the respiratory and circulatory systems by activities which require only a modest increase of oxygen intake and so can be maintained."

The tricky issue is determining how much aerobic exercise is just enough to insure health benefits without increasing the chances that you'll injure yourself or have a medical emergency.

Steven N. Blair, director of epidemiology at The Cooper Institute for Aerobics Research, and researchers from other medical institutions (including the Centers for Disease Control, Stanford University, and the University of Wisconsin) examined this issue in depth.[6,7,8] They reviewed the findings of many exercise studies and identified an ideal upper and lower limit of exercise. Although more research is needed, there does appear to be a just-right level of exercise, which is far less than the strenuous workouts that exercise enthusiasts engage in as a matter of course. In the language of exercise physiologists:

> Exercise training that results in a weekly energy expenditure of between *10 and 20 calories per kilogram of body weight** is likely to bring about major health benefits.[6,7] Twenty calories is the upper limit necessary from a health promotion standpoint— energy expenditures above this level do not appear to provide substantially more benefit.[6] The lower limit of 10 calories is necessary to insure effectiveness,[7] although lesser amounts are still likely to be of some benefit.[9]

These conclusions about energy expenditure form the mathematical basis of the Health Points System described in the next chapter. Most patients would find it difficult to figure out how much exercise is needed to expend 10 to 20 calories per kilogram of body weight. Our Health Points System transforms these seemingly complicated recommendations into a practical, easy-to-follow method of assessing the effectiveness of your exercise program. So if you're concerned about the complexity of calculating your weekly energy expenditure,

---

*1 kilogram = approximately 2.2 pounds. 1 calorie = approximately 4.2 kilojoules.

stop worrying—our Health Points System will take care of this for you.

Here are two examples: Mark Davis weighed 202 pounds (92 kilograms) when he first arrived at The Cooper Aerobics Center. So he needed to gradually build up to a weekly energy expenditure of between 920 (92 × 10) and 1,840 (92 × 20) calories during exercise. Linda Stone weighed 125 pounds (57 kilograms). Her target weekly energy expenditure during exercise was 570 (57 × 10) to 1,140 (57 × 20) calories.

Factors That Determine Energy Expenditure

Weekly energy expenditure during exercise depends largely on four factors: the type, frequency, intensity, and duration of your exercise sessions. Discuss these four factors with your doctor when you meet to tailor a safe and effective weekly exercise regimen for you. Keeping both your medical condition and personal preferences in mind, your doctor should help you do the following:

- Choose a suitable aerobic exercise.
- Decide on the number of times you should work out each week.
- Determine the appropriate exercise intensity.
- Establish how long each exercise session should last.

It's important for you to understand how the last three items intertwine. They're embodied in the concept of FIT, which is an acronym for **F**requency, **I**ntensity, and **T**ime. If you exercise regularly, you're undoubtedly familiar with this notion already. *Frequency* refers to how often you exercise. *Intensity* refers to how hard you exert yourself. *Time* refers to each exercise session's duration. An equation showing their interrelationship would look like this:

$$\textbf{F}\text{requency} + \textbf{I}\text{ntensity} + \textbf{T}\text{ime} = \text{Caloric Energy Expenditure}$$
$$= \text{Health Benefit}$$

If the amount on the right side of the equation (caloric energy expenditure and health benefit) remains constant and you cut down on one or two elements on the left side of the equation, the third element on the left side must increase to make up the difference. For example, if you exercise at a low to moderate intensity 3 days a week, each session may have to last a relatively long time to substantially benefit your health. You may choose instead to exercise at the same low to moderate intensity but for a shorter length of time each session.

In this instance, you'll need to increase the number of times per week that you exercise to achieve the desired weekly energy expenditure.

Here are my recommendations concerning each of these factors:

Frequency.   I recommend 3 to 5 days per week as the ideal exercise schedule for people with Type I or Type II diabetes and for those without diabetes. Less is unlikely to produce significant health improvements; more predisposes you to musculoskeletal injuries.

Today, most experts believe that it's not practical for people with Type I diabetes to attempt to significantly improve their blood-glucose control with daily exercise. But the experts do believe exercise can increase the body's insulin sensitivity in both Type I and Type II diabetes patients. It's always best to space your workouts evenly throughout the week, with no more than a day or two of rest between sessions, and this is especially important for people with diabetes. Why? Because a single bout of exercise increases your insulin sensitivity, but the effect lasts only 2 or 3 days at the very most. Even after many months of regular exercise, your insulin sensitivity may return to pretraining levels after as few as 3 days of inactivity.[10]

Time or Duration.   The higher the intensity or frequency, the shorter the time needed to attain the desired weekly energy expenditure. For most diabetes patients, workouts of 30 to 45 minutes are ideal. Moderate-intensity aerobic exercise of longer duration is preferable to high-intensity exercise of shorter duration for diabetes patients for these reasons: it lessens the risk of training-related medical complications; it is probably more beneficial for blood-glucose control; and the average person is more likely to enjoy moderate workouts. Longer, moderate workouts are particularly important if weight loss is a goal because they promote fat loss while reducing the risk of musculoskeletal injuries.

Workouts of 30 to 45 minutes of continuous aerobic exercise should be the eventual goal for most of you. But if your fitness level is very low, you might want to consider a viable alternative documented by Stanford University researchers. They found that three 10-minute exercise sessions spread throughout the day may yield fitness gains similar to one 30-minute session.[11]

Remember that these recommendations on duration do not include the warm-up and cool-down periods, which should open and close each aerobics session. Take at least 5 minutes to ease into aerobics, going from a low intensity and slowly building up to your peak target intensity. Also, reduce your exercise intensity gradually for 5 minutes at the end of your workout.

Intensity.   The notion that you must exercise at high intensities to derive health benefits is a fallacy. In short, the "no pain, no gain" axiom is wrong. It's also a dangerous idea for people with diabetes who have chronic cardiac, vascular, or neurological complications. Fortunately, optimal health benefits can be derived with a minimum of risk by exercising at a moderate rather than a high intensity.

There are several ways to quantify exercise intensity, and I'll discuss three: metabolic equivalent units (METs), heart rate, and perceived exertion.

How to Quantify Exercise Intensity

METs.   One MET is the amount of oxygen your body consumes for energy production each minute you're at rest. If you're engaged in an activity corresponding to 5 METs, this means that your body is taking up and using five times more oxygen than it did at rest. It now needs that much oxygen to fuel your working muscles, so they can produce enough energy. I'll discuss METs later in this chapter when I explain how to select an appropriate speed or work rate for the first weeks of a walking or stationary cycling exercise program.

Heart Rate.   This is perhaps the most widely used and helpful way to target exercise intensity. It's based on the principle that there's a direct relationship between the increase in your body's oxygen uptake during exertion and the increase in your heart rate.

I advise my patients with diabetes to exercise at an intensity that raises the heart rate above 60% of their maximal heart rate but no higher than 85%. That range spans 25 percentage points. In fact, other experts and I have found that an exercise heart rate in the range of 60% to 75% of the maximal heart rate is ideal for most diabetes patients.[12]

What's your maximal heart rate? The figure varies between individuals. Your maximal heart rate is the highest heart rate that you can attain during exercise without developing any significant cardiovascular abnormalities.

The most accurate way to determine your maximal heart rate is to have a treadmill or cycle exercise test. In medical jargon, it's called a *symptom-limited maximal exercise test with electrocardiogram (ECG) monitoring*; the term *symptom-limited* simply means that you exercise until you cannot continue because you are too fatigued or because you develop ECG or other abnormalities that indicate to your physician that the test should be stopped. I strongly advocate that all my adult diabetes patients take an exercise test. The test will enable your doctor to tell you the highest heart rate you can achieve without developing any cardiovascular abnormalities. *This is the value you should use as your maximal heart rate.*

Both Mark and Linda had exercise tests. Mark's maximal heart rate was 165 beats per minute; Linda's was 184 beats per minute. If you don't have a test, you can use the following formula to *estimate* your maximal heart rate:

For all women and sedentary men:
220 minus your age in years   = Estimated Maximal
                                               Heart Rate

For conditioned men:
205 minus one-half your age in years   = Estimated Maximal
                                               Heart Rate

Your estimated value may differ from your actual rate. For example, Mark at age 46 had an estimated maximal heart rate of 174 beats per minute (220 – 46 = 174). At age 29, Linda's estimated maximal heart rate was 191 beats per minute (220 – 29 = 191) before she began our supervised exercise program. Note that Mark's actual maximal heart rate was 165, slightly lower than his estimate. Linda's actual rate (184) was also lower.

These formulas are invalid for people taking medications, such as beta blockers, that slow down the heart rate. They're also invalid for those with autonomic neuropathy, for this can also slow down the heart rate. And for safety reasons, I caution people who know they have heart disease to ignore these formulas, whether or not they're taking medication.

Training Target Heart Rate Zone.   Once you know your maximal heart rate (either estimated using the formula or determined precisely by an exercise test), it's *easy* to determine the exercise intensity levels you should stay within. As I mentioned previously, I recommend that you push your heart rate above 60% of your maximal heart rate but no higher than 75% (and definitely not above 85%). This is your *training target heart rate zone*, which you can calculate by multiplying your maximal heart rate by the lower limit of 60% (or 0.6) and the upper limit of 75% (or 0.75).

Using Mark's actual maximal heart rate of 165, he calculated a lower limit of 99 beats per minute ($165 \times 0.6 = 99$) and an upper limit of 124 beats per minute ($165 \times 0.75 = 124$). Linda's training target heart rate zone was between 110 ($184 \times 0.6 = 110$) and 138 ($184 \times 0.75 = 138$) beats per minute.

This zone is important. Studies show that exercise performed at an intensity lower than 60% may net you some health benefits but is unlikely to substantially increase your fitness level.[3] And you need to exceed this level to insure that you're increasing your body's insulin sensitivity, a key goal of exercise for persons with diabetes. If you don't exceed the 60% mark, you'll also probably have to lengthen each session to well over an hour to attain the recommended weekly energy expenditure. On the other hand, if you're under time pressure and you can only work out a maximum of 3 days a week or for short durations when you do find time, you'll need to exercise near the upper limit of your training target heart rate zone to gain any appreciable health benefit.

Remember it's crucial never to exceed the 85% upper limit (the only exceptions are competitive athletes). During high-intensity exercise, your blood-glucose level increases; it doesn't decrease, as you might think.[13] Also, in people with cardiovascular complications, intensities above the 85% limit increase the risk for triggering cardiovascular problems during exercise.

Using Heart Rate to Guide Intensity.   For novice exercisers, the questions and answers that follow provide more insight into how to use your heart rate as a guide to your exercise intensity:

• *How do I measure my heart rate during exercise?* The same way you'd do it at rest—by taking your pulse. (See Appendix A.)

• *How often during exercise should I calculate my heart rate?* Initially, you may need to check your heart rate as often as every 5 minutes. But once you are familiar with your appropriate exercise intensity, you may need to do it only a few times each workout. I generally recommend that you check your rate at the following times:

1. *Before starting to exercise.* If it is above 100 beats per minute and remains this high after 15 minutes or so of rest, don't exercise at all. Check your blood-glucose level to make sure that you do not have hypoglycemia; a rapid heart rate is a warning sign of hypoglycemia.
2. *After you complete your warm-up.* If, at this point, your heart rate is above the upper limit you have set, slow down

until it drops below this limit. You performed your warm-up at too high an intensity. Start off slower next time.

3. *After you've been exercising at your peak intensity for about 5 minutes.* If it is above your upper limit, slow down and recheck it within 5 minutes.

4. *When you stop the aerobic phase and begin your cool-down.*

5. *When you complete your cool-down.* If your heart rate isn't below 100 beats per minute, rest until it reaches this level. Only then should you take a shower or drive off in your car.

- *Can I rely on a portable heart rate monitor instead of checking my heart rate manually?* Commercially available meters are generally worn on the chest and provide continual monitoring of your heart rate by transmitting electrical signals to a special wristwatch or computer that's also worn on your chest. Usually, you can program your heart rate limit into the device, and it will set off an alarm if you exceed it. Provided you purchase a reliable model, such monitors can be helpful, but they're certainly not a necessity. I suggest you consult a member of your health-care team before buying one. Ask which type he or she thinks is most accurate. Then before you purchase a specific one, ask that team member to help you verify its accuracy while you're wearing it.

Perceived Exertion. One of the simplest ways to quantify exercise intensity is to use the scale in Table 3.1 (see page 50). Named after the Swedish exercise physiologist Gunnar Borg who developed it in the early 1950s, the Borg scale helps you judge your exercise intensity based on your on-the-spot perception of how difficult the exercise feels.[14] This *rating of perceived exertion* (RPE) is outlined on a scale from 6 to 20, which you consult as you exercise. If you're exerting yourself at a level that you feel is fairly strenuous, you might assign your effort an RPE of 13. When you reach the all-out huffing-and-puffing stage, you'd choose a much higher rating of about 17.

Generally, an RPE of 12 to 13 corresponds to an exercise intensity of 60% to 75% of the maximal heart rate. In other words, the 12-to-13 RPE range corresponds to your training target heart rate zone, which you should aim for during the aerobic portion of your workouts. Unless you're a competitive athlete, never exceed a score of 15, even if your heart rate is below your limit.

Basic Aerobic Exercises to Get You Started

Aerobic exercises *don't* require excessive speed or strength, but they *do* place demands on your cardiovascular system. Examples of aerobic exercises are brisk walking, running, swimming, cross-country skiing, and cycling.

Anaerobic means "without oxygen." Sprinting is an anaerobic activity. It involves an all-out burst of effort and relies on metabolic processes that do not require oxygen for energy production. Such processes cause fatigue quickly.

Aerobic exercise is far better than anaerobic exercise for people with diabetes for these reasons: Energy expenditure is related to how much oxygen your working muscles use during exercise. Aerobic exercise uses up more oxygen than anaerobic exercise. Also, because it's more moderate and you can do it longer, aerobic exercise allows you to expend far more energy than anaerobic exercise. And when you exercise aerobically, you can better monitor your heart rate and keep it within your prescribed limit. Anaerobic exercise is more likely to push your heart rate above that limit, which can be dangerous if you have cardiovascular disease. Anaerobic exercise is also likely to raise rather than lower your blood-glucose level.

The aerobic exercises I most commonly recommend for diabetes patients beginning an exercise program are walking, jogging, and stationary cycling. Each has its pluses and minuses.

Walking. Most experts, including me, consider walking one of the most appropriate aerobic activities for diabetes patients.[15] The intensity is easy to control, so even many people with chronic diabetes complications can walk and get the desired conditioning effect. It's simple and requires no special skill, setting, or equipment other than a good pair of shoes. It's also one of the least likely activities to cause musculoskeletal problems. And in a recent study, Tom R. Thomas and Ben R. Londeree found that at fast speeds the energy expenditure for walking approaches that for jogging.[16]

Jogging. The advantages of jogging are similar to those for walking. The catch is that jogging generally requires greater exertion, or intensity, than walking, often causing your heart rate to exceed your limit. Also, it may increase your risk for musculoskeletal problems, foot complications if you have peripheral neuropathy, and eye complications if you have preproliferative or proliferative retinopathy. But if you're enthusiastic about jogging, despite the greater risks, I recommend you begin with a walking program and then a walk/jog regimen before trying jogging.

Stationary Cycling. Busy people love this activity. While pedaling away on your stationary cycle (also known as a *cycle ergometer*), you can do other things—read or watch TV, for example. Stationary cycling gives you no excuse should the weather make outdoor cycling impossible, and it causes less wear and tear on the musculoskeletal system than jogging. Moreover, because it is a low-impact activity, it's ideally suited to patients with retinopathy.

Some stationary cycles, such as the Schwinn Air-Dyne, help you expend more energy by working your arms and legs simultaneously. You pump your legs up and down while you move your arms forward and back. The result is a more thorough upper and lower body work-out. I recommend these cycle ergometers for my patients, especially those who use their arms a lot at work or for recreation.

Arm-Cycle Ergometry. This is another alternative for patients who use their arms a lot. People with leg amputations or other problems that prevent them from using their legs during exercise (such as paraplegia, foot ulcers, and peripheral vascular disease) will also benefit from arm-cycle ergometry.

Outdoor Cycling. In my opinion, outdoor cycling is far more enjoyable and exhilarating than pedaling away indoors. The disadvantage over a stationary workout is that roads tend to go up and down. An unexpected incline could cause your heart rate to rise too high. Also, too many downhill stretches and delays at stoplights may lessen your energy expenditure so much that you must work out longer to meet your energy expenditure goal. Then, of course, there is the problem of traffic and the danger it poses. But if you can manage these drawbacks, outdoor cycling is great.

PUTTING ON THOSE WALKING SHOES
AND VENTURING FORTH

Here I offer you guidelines on initiating a walking, walk/jog, or stationary cycling exercise program. I recommend these forms of exercise to sedentary adult diabetes patients because they're a good way to slowly ease into the routine of regular exercise.

After you've completed an introductory 8 to 12 weeks or so following one of these programs, you'll be ready to start trying to earn the 50 to 100 exercise health points I'll discuss in the next chapter. Please note that these programs are intended as a guideline. Your individual circumstances may require you to progress more slowly.

Beginning Walking Program

Walking is a wonderful way to get moving down the road to optimal health. But before you begin, you need to know your maximal MET value so you can estimate the speed (in mph or kph) at which you should walk during the first 8 weeks. Your maximal MET value depends on your fitness level. If you've had an exercise test (which I urge all diabetes patients to do), your doctor can provide you with your maximal MET value. If not, err on the side of caution. Start at a comfortable speed that does not exceed what's recommended for a person with a maximal MET value of 6. Whether or not you know your maximal MET value, I strongly advise against exceeding 75% of your maximal heart rate and an RPE of 13 during these initial weeks. Table 3.2 on page 51 shows you what your estimated beginning walking speed should be. Using this table, Mark Davis, whose maximal MET value was 6, started his walking program at a speed of about 3.4 mph, or 5.4 kph. The box on page 51 shows you what your walking program will look like in terms of each workout's duration and frequency.

A Follow-Up Walk/Jog Program

Don't try jogging until you've followed a walking regimen for at least 6 weeks, ideally 12 weeks. In your walking program, you should be walking at speeds in excess of 4 mph just before you graduate to jogging. If you're walking at a slower rate, you might as well stay with walking. Here are some pointers:

- When you start to jog, do so at a speed no faster than that at which you currently walk.
- As always, warm up and cool down for 5 minutes each. For the warm-up phase, walk briskly and try to gradually raise your heart rate to within at least 20 beats per minute of your target heart rate. On completing your jog, gradually reduce your speed to a slow walk over a 5-minute period.

The boxes on pages 52 and 53 show what your walk/jog program will look like in terms of each workout's duration and frequency.

Beginning Stationary Cycling Program

If indoor cycling is more to your liking than walking, that's fine. It's an excellent form of exercise.

Before you begin, you should know your maximal MET value and your weight in either pounds or kilograms (in the boxes that follow, choose the weight closest to yours). If you haven't had an exercise test and don't know your maximal MET value, start out at a comfortable work rate that does not exceed that recommended for a person with a maximal MET value of 6. Whether you know your maximal MET value or not, I strongly advise against exceeding 75% of your maximal heart rate and an RPE of 13 during these initial weeks. Table 3.3 on page 54 shows your estimated beginning work rate for a stationary cycling program. Linda Stone, who weighed 125 pounds and had a maximal MET value of 8, began her cycling program at 67 watts. Duration and frequency recommendations for the first 8 weeks of your cycling program are shown in the box on page 54.

Beginning Schwinn Air-Dyne Cycling Program

A second form of indoor cycling, which works both your arms and legs, is the Schwinn Air-Dyne, another good choice for beginning a regular exercise habit. Table 3.4 on page 55 shows how to estimate your work load for the first 8 weeks. If you don't know your maximal MET value, start at a comfortable work load that corresponds to a maximal MET value no higher than 6. Whether you know your maximal MET value or not, I strongly advise against exceeding 75% of your maximal heart rate and an RPE of 13 during these initial weeks. If you weigh 154 pounds (70 kilograms) and have a maximal MET value of 7, you would see by looking at Table 3.4 that you should cycle at a work load of 1.3.

The box on page 55 shows duration and frequency recommendations for your Schwinn Air-Dyne routine. There are several other superb cycle ergometers that enable you to work your arms and legs simultaneously. If you prefer to use one of them, these recommendations are equally applicable.

Beginning Program of Combined Walking and Stationary Cycling Using the Schwinn Air-Dyne

Some people get bored doing the same exercise day after day. For such people, I've devised an 8-week regimen that combines walking with cycling on the Schwinn Air-Dyne. This combination will also help reduce your risk of injury.

My guidelines for walking and Schwinn Air-Dyne workouts also apply to the combined program. Estimate your starting walking speed and Schwinn Air-Dyne work load for the first 8 weeks of this program using Tables 3.2 and 3.4.

You may start with either activity. As always, warm up for 5 minutes. After completing the first activity, proceed immediately to the other one—another warm-up is not needed. Upon completing the second activity, cool down for 5 minutes. The duration and frequency recommendations are shown in the box on page 56.

THAT ALL-IMPORTANT TRAINING LOG

I encourage all of our diabetes patients to keep track of their exercise efforts, at least in the beginning, via a training log. A diary is a good idea because it provides you and your doctor with helpful data. Moreover, it will help you be consistent and stay on track with your exercise program. Two empty training log pages follow—the first for people with Type II diabetes and the second for people on insulin therapy. Make a number of photocopies of the appropriate page and put them in a loose-leaf notebook. Fill in a page after each day's exercise.

DAILY EXERCISE TRAINING LOG

Date _____   Time of day _____   Body weight _____

Where I worked out _____

Resting pulse _____

Pre-exercise blood glucose (if measured) _____

Post-exercise blood glucose (if measured) _____

Duration of stretching and strengthening portion
   of my workout _____

Pulse rate after stretching and strengthening portion
   of my workout (in beats per minute) _____

Aerobic portion of workout

   Type of exercise _____

   Duration (in minutes) _____

   Distance covered or work rate/load _____

   Highest heart rate _____

   Borg RPE (at most intense part of workout) _____

   Any symptoms experienced _____

Enjoyment rating   _____ 1 Very unenjoyable

                   _____ 2 Unenjoyable

                   _____ 3 Somewhat unenjoyable

                   _____ 4 Enjoyable

                   _____ 5 Very enjoyable

Health points earned (see chapter 4) _____

DAILY EXERCISE TRAINING LOG

Month / Day	Diet/drug therapy														
	Pre-breakfast		Pre-breakfast insulin			Pre-lunch		Pre-lunch insulin	Pre-supper		Pre-supper insulin			Pre-bedtime		Pre-bedtime snack
	BG	Ket	Sh	Int	Long	BG	Ket		BG	Ket	Sh	Int	Long	BG	Ket	

KEY TO ABBREVIATIONS:

BG = blood glucose
Ket = ketones
Sh = short-acting
Int = intermediate-acting
Long = long-acting
Food = number of food exchanges or grams of carbohydrate or calories ingested
Peak HR = highest heart rate during workout
RPE = Borg rating of perceived exertion

FOR PEOPLE ON INSULIN THERAPY

								Exercise training				
Pre-BG	Pre-ket	Pre-food	Time of day	During BG	During food	Post-BG	Post-food	Enjoyment rating*	Exercise time	Distance or work rate/load	Peak HR	RPE
Type of exercise	Comments								Health points score			
Type of exercise	Comments								Health points score			
Type of exercise	Comments								Health points score			
Type of exercise	Comments								Health points score			
Type of exercise	Comments								Health points score			
Type of exercise	Comments								Health points score			
Type of exercise	Comments								Health points score			
										Week's total health points		

*ENJOYMENT RATING SCORES

1–very unenjoyable
2–unenjoyable
3–somewhat unenjoyable
4–enjoyable
5–very enjoyable

Table 3.1
Borg Perceived Exertion Scale

The original Borg system for rating physical exertion is based on an open-ended scale running from 6 (equal to exertion at rest) to 20 (extreme effort).

Rating of perceived exertion or RPE	Verbal description of RPE
6	
7	Very, very light
8	
9	Very light
10	
11	Fairly light
12	
13	Somewhat hard
14	
15	Hard
16	
17	Very hard
18	
19	Very, very hard
20	

Note. From G.A. Borg, "Psychophysical Bases of Perceived Exertion," *Medicine and Science in Sports and Exercise, 14*, pp. 377-387, 1982, © by The American College of Sports Medicine. Reprinted by permission.

Table 3.2
Estimated Speed at Which to Begin a Walking Program

Maximal MET value	Estimated walking speed (miles per hour)	Estimated walking speed (kilometers per hour)
4	1.8 mph	2.9 kph
5	2.6 mph	4.2 kph
6	3.4 mph	5.4 kph
7 and above	4 mph	6.4 kph

Walking Program		
Week	**Duration per session**	**Frequency per week**
1	10 minutes	3-5 times
2	15 minutes	3-5 times
3	20 minutes	3-5 times
4	25 minutes	3-5 times
5	30 minutes	3-5 times
6	35 minutes	3-5 times
7	40 minutes	3-5 times
8	45 minutes	3-5 times
9 and onward	It's time to start earning those 50 to 100 health points a week. Keep your exercise time at 45 minutes per session and gradually increase your speed until you exceed 60% of your maximal heart rate (if you are not doing so yet). If this does not result in the desired weekly energy expenditure using the health points charts in chapter 4,* do one or more of the following: Try exercising within the upper range of your target heart rate zone, exercise more frequently, or increase the duration of each exercise session.	

*At fast speeds, the energy you expend for walking approaches that for jogging. Therefore, for speeds of 4 mph (or 6.4 kph) or faster, I recommend that you use our jogging chart in chapter 4 to calculate your health points.

Walk-Jog Program		
Week	**Duration per session**	**Frequency per week**
1	*20 minutes total*—Walk 4.5 min, jog 0.5 min, walk 4.5 min, jog 0.5 min, walk 4.5 min, jog 0.5 min, walk 4.5 min, jog 0.5 min*	3-5 times
2	*20 minutes total*—Walk 4 min, jog 1 min, walk 4 min, jog 1 min, walk 4 min, jog 1 min, walk 4 min, jog 1 min*	3-5 times
3	*20 minutes total*—Walk 3 min, jog 2 min, walk 3 min, jog 2 min, walk 3 min, jog 2 min, walk 3 min, jog 2 min*	3-5 times
4	*20 minutes total*—Walk 2 min, jog 3 min, walk 2 min, jog 3 min, walk 2 min, jog 3 min, walk 2 min, jog 3 min*	3-5 times
5	*20 minutes total*—Walk 5 min, jog 5 min, walk 5 min, jog 5 min*	3-5 times
6	*20 minutes total*—Walk 4 min, jog 6 min, walk 4 min, jog 6 min*	3-5 times
7	*20 minutes total*—Walk 3 min, jog 7 min, walk 3 min, jog 7 min*	3-5 times

(Cont.)

Walk-Jog Program (Continued)		
Week	**Duration per session**	**Frequency per week**
8	*20 minutes total*—Jog 10 min, walk 10 min*	3-5 times
9	*20 minutes total*—Jog 12 min, walk 8 min*	3-5 times
10	*20 minutes total*—Jog 15 min, walk 5 min*	3-5 times
11	*20 minutes total*—Jog 17 min, walk 3 min*	3-5 times
12	*20 minutes total*—Jog 20 min*	3-5 times
13 and onward	By the time you reach this point, you are likely to have exceeded 60% of your maximal heart rate, and you've possibly attained your desired weekly energy expenditure—100 health points per week —using the health points charts in chapter 4.* If so, just keep following week 12's regimen. If, on the other hand, you haven't been able to exceed 60% of your maximal heart rate, increase your speed. If that does not result in 100 weekly health points, do one or more of the following: Try exercising within the upper range of your target heart rate zone, exercise more frequently, or increase the duration of each exercise session.	

*You may find that you are below your desired weekly energy expenditure during the early weeks of this walk-jog effort. You can compensate by walking longer at the end of the jogging phase, before starting your cool-down. Use the jogging chart in chapter 4 when calculating your health points for your walk-jog program.

Table 3.3
Estimated Work Rate at Which to Begin a Stationary Cycling (Legs Only) Program

	Work rate (watts)					
Maximal MET value	Body weight = 110 lb (50 kg)	Body weight = 132 lb (60 kg)	Body weight = 154 lb (70 kg)	Body weight = 176 lb (80 kg)	Body weight = 198 lb (90 kg)	Body weight = 220 lb (100 kg)
4	20	25	29	33	37	41
5	29	35	41	47	53	58
6	38	46	53	61	68	76
7	47	56	65	75	84	93
8 and above	55	67	78	89	100	111

Stationary Cycling Program

Week	Duration per session	Frequency per week
1	7.5 minutes	3-5 times
2	10 minutes	3-5 times
3	12.5 minutes	3-5 times
4	15 minutes	3-5 times
5	17.5 minutes	3-5 times
6	20 minutes	3-5 times
7	25 minutes	3-5 times
8	30 minutes	3-5 times
9 and onward	It's time to start earning those 50 to 100 health points a week. Keep your exercise time at 30 minutes per session and gradually increase your work rate until you exceed 60% of your maximal heart rate (if you are not doing so yet). If this does not result in the desired weekly energy expenditure using the health points charts in chapter 4, do one or more of the following: Try exercising within the upper range of your target heart rate zone, exercise more frequently, or increase the duration of each exercise session.	

Table 3.4
Estimated Work Load at Which to Begin a Schwinn Air-Dyne Cycling Program

	Work load					
Maximal MET value	Body weight = 110 lb (50 kg)	Body weight = 132 lb (60 kg)	Body weight = 154 lb (70 kg)	Body weight = 176 lb (80 kg)	Body weight = 198 lb (90 kg)	Body weight = 220 lb (100 kg)
4	.4	.5	.6	.7	.7	.8
5	.6	.7	.8	.9	1.1	1.2
6	.8	.9	1.1	1.2	1.4	1.5
7	.9	1.1	1.3	1.5	1.7	1.9
8 and above	1.1	1.3	1.6	1.8	2	2.2

Schwinn Air-Dyne Program		
Week	**Duration per session**	**Frequency per week**
1	7.5 minutes	3-5 times
2	10 minutes	3-5 times
3	12.5 minutes	3-5 times
4	15 minutes	3-5 times
5	17.5 minutes	3-5 times
6	20 minutes	3-5 times
7	25 minutes	3-5 times
8	30 minutes	3-5 times
9 and onward	It's time to start earning those 50 to 100 health points a week. Keep your exercise time at 30 minutes per session and gradually increase your work load until you exceed 60% of your maximal heart rate (if you are not doing so yet). If this does not result in the desired weekly energy expenditure using the health points charts in chapter 4, do one or more of the following: Try exercising within the upper range of your target heart rate zone, exercise more frequently, or increase the duration of each exercise session.	

Combined Walking and Schwinn Air-Dyne Program

	Duration per session		
	---	---	---
Week	Walking	Schwinn Air-Dyne	Frequency per week
1	5 minutes	5 minutes	3-5 times
2	7.5 minutes	7.5 minutes	3-5 times
3	10 minutes	10 minutes	3-5 times
4	12.5 minutes	12.5 minutes	3-5 times
5	15 minutes	15 minutes	3-5 times
6	17.5 minutes	17.5 minutes	3-5 times
7	20 minutes	20 minutes	3-5 times
8	22.5 minutes	22.5 minutes	3-5 times
9 and onward	It's time to start earning those 50 to 100 health points a week. Keep the combined exercise time at 45 minutes per session and gradually increase the intensity until you exceed 60% of your maximal heart rate (if you're not doing so yet). If this does not result in the desired weekly energy expenditure using the health points charts in chapter 4, do one or more of the following: Try exercising within the upper range of your target heart rate zone, exercise more frequently, or increase the duration of each exercise session.		

Chapter 3
Prescription

☐ Start your exercise program slowly and progress gradually.

☐ Include both a warm-up and a cool-down of at least 5 minutes' duration in each exercise session.

☐ Do stretching and, unless contraindicated, aerobic exercises three to five times each week.

☐ Include muscle-strengthening exercises in your routines two to three times each week.

☐ Structure the aerobic portion of your workout so that it is eventually 15 to 60 minutes long.

☐ Aim for an exercise intensity that raises your heart rate to between 60% and 75% of your maximal value and elicits an RPE of 12 to 13 during the aerobic portion of your workout.

☐ Don't exceed 85% of your maximal heart rate or an RPE of 15 at any point in your workout.

☐ Exercise your options: Choose aerobic exercises that are convenient to do.

☐ Keep track of your exercise efforts in a training diary.

Chapter 4

The Health Points System: Insuring Maximum Health Benefits With Minimum Risk

In trying to motivate our diabetes patients to follow my exercise prescription, I'm always juggling several responsibilities. First, as a physician, I must educate patients adequately so their excuse can never be "I didn't understand." Then I have to alert them to the seriousness of their condition and the risks involved in exercise without leaving them with the feeling it's hopeless. And, most importantly, I must make them understand that drugs and medical care can go only so far in making them well. They must do the rest by making positive lifestyle changes, including adhering to a regular exercise program.

The impetus for our Health Points System grew out of these needs, especially the need to make you, the patient, responsible for your own health. With the Health Points System, you have, for the first time, a way to chart how effective your exercise program is likely to be in promoting your health.*

Our Health Points System was designed so that patients will do just enough exercise to gain optimal health benefits without exerting themselves to the point where exercise becomes risky. Our system helps you strike a balance between effectiveness and safety.

HOW THE HEALTH POINTS SYSTEM WORKS

Our system is based on the number of calories people expend during exercise, which varies according to weight. In chapter 3, I discussed what doctors and exercise physiologists have learned about aerobic exercise and its effects on health. Let's review this key finding:

> Aerobic exercise performed for 15 to 60 minutes per workout 3 to 5 days each week at an intensity that raises the heart rate to between 60% and 85% of the maximal value will result in an energy expenditure that brings about the desired health benefits.

Here's how the Health Points System works. If you're a novice exerciser, follow one of the beginning exercise programs outlined in chapter 3 and gradually work up to an appropriate level of exertion over 8 weeks or so. Although you can start using the Weekly Health Points Exercise Tally Sheet (see page 61) during this time, do not specifically try to earn 50 to 100 health points until you reach Week 9. Depending on the severity of any diabetes complications you may have, it may take you much longer than this to earn the desired points. That's fine. Be patient.

In all aspects of life, we humans like to know where we stand in our endeavors. We like to get report cards. Our Health Points System is a kind of report card on your exercise program. Only you fill it out, not a doctor or a teacher. Our system enables you to quantify one constructive lifestyle change—namely, regular aerobic exercise—that you can easily undertake to improve your health and reduce your risk of developing diabetes complications. It gives you a way to chart your progress so you can see, in black and white, what you are accomplishing and where you stand.

---

*Those of you with no diabetes complications have the option of following Ken Cooper's well-known Aerobic Points System instead of our Health Points System. He describes it fully in *The Aerobics Program for Total Well-Being.*[1]

WEEKLY HEALTH POINTS EXERCISE TALLY SHEET

Your Weekly Goal: To earn between 50 and 100 health points each week, which corresponds to an expenditure of 10 to 20 calories per kilogram (2.2 pounds) of body weight per week. Exceeding this upper limit does not provide substantially more health benefit; thus you should keep your weekly health points total at, or very near, 100. To gain optimal benefit, you should earn your weekly quota of points across at least 3 workouts.

To find out how many health points you earned during an exercise session, simply use the chart (see Tables 4.1-4.5, pages 72-79) that corresponds to the form of aerobic exercise you're doing and fill in the results below:

Monday	Tuesday	Wednesday	Thursday	Friday	Saturday	Sunday	Total weekly health points
___ pt. +	___ pt. +	___ pt. +	___ pt. +	___ pt. +	___ pt. +	___ pt. =	___ pt. (100 pt. maximum)

INTERPRETING THE EFFECTIVENESS OF YOUR WEEKLY EXERCISE EFFORT*

100 health points from exercise	Ideal. *You couldn't do better!*
70-99 health points from exercise	Very good. *Be proud of yourself.*
50-69 health points from exercise	Good. *But you could do better.*
20-49 health points from exercise	Fair. *Try a bit harder.*
10-19 health points from exercise	Poor. *But it's better than nothing.*
Less than 10 health points from exercise	Very poor. *Come on, now.*

*If your clinical condition is such that you are unable to attain the desired weekly number of health points, please ignore this interpretation. Be proud of whatever progress you are able to make.

Our Health Points System is a lifelong program for attaining and maintaining optimal well-being. But some of you with severe diabetes complications—or those of you who have musculoskeletal disorders such as arthritis—may not be able to attain the desired weekly number of health points. Don't worry or become discouraged. If you do some type of aerobic exercise—even an exercise for which I don't provide health points charts—for a minimum of 15 minutes at least 3 days a week, you'll derive important health benefits. Rather than trying to meet goals that may be unrealistic given your circumstances, be proud of what progress you can make. Also, keep in mind that the effectiveness categories in the Weekly Health Points Exercise Tally Sheet are not applicable to persons whose clinical condition (as opposed to factors such as a lack of interest or desire) prevents them from attaining the recommended weekly health points.

HOW TO USE
THE HEALTH POINTS CHARTS

The only way to accurately measure energy expenditure during exercise is through laboratory testing. There, technicians utilize sophisticated equipment to determine the exact amount of oxygen the body uses during a workout. Our health points are based on numerous exercise studies performed in such laboratories.

The health points charts at the end of this chapter (Tables 4.1-4.4) show you how to calculate health points for walking, jogging, stationary cycling (legs only), and the Schwinn Air-Dyne (beginning exercise programs for these activities were outlined in chapter 3). We could formulate charts for these forms of exercise because (a) they don't require much skill and (b) outstanding research data are available on them.

If you're exercising on equipment that gives you a readout of the calories you've expended, you can easily convert that number to health points. First, obtain your conversion number by dividing your body weight in pounds by 11 (or if your body weight is in kilograms, divide it by 5). Then divide the calories expended by your conversion number to obtain your health points. For example, if the readout number is 120 calories and you weigh 165 pounds (75 kilograms), you've earned 8 health points (165 pounds ÷ 11 = 75 kilograms ÷ 5 = 15 and 120 calories ÷ 15 = 8 health points).

To determine your health points for walking and jogging, you need to know the distance you covered (to convert kilometers to miles,

Other aerobic choices

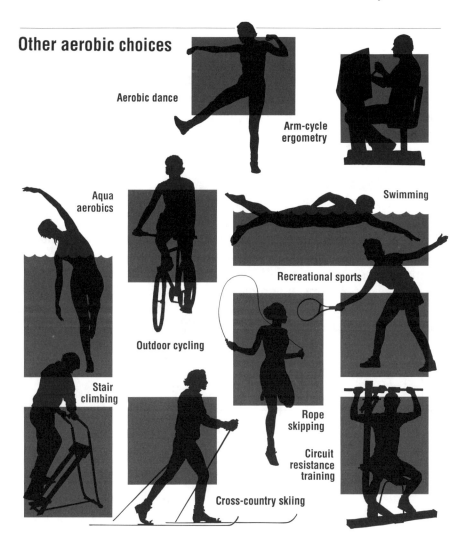

Aerobic dance

Arm-cycle ergometry

Aqua aerobics

Swimming

Outdoor cycling

Recreational sports

Stair climbing

Rope skipping

Circuit resistance training

Cross-country skiing

divide by 1.6) and the time it took you. If you have access to a measured running track, figuring the distance will pose no problem. Otherwise you might want to buy a pedometer or use your car's odometer to stake out a stretch of road to use as a track. You'll need a watch with a second hand or a stopwatch to accurately time your sessions.

To find your health points on the charts for stationary cycling (legs only) and the Schwinn Air-Dyne, you'll need to know the duration of your workout, your work rate (wattage) or work load (for the Schwinn Air-Dyne), and your weight (to convert kilograms to pounds, multiply by 2.2).

To show you how easy the Health Points System is to use, on this page and the next are some examples from Mark Davis's and Linda Stone's training diaries. At the time, Mark weighed 187 pounds (85 kilograms) and Linda weighed 125 pounds (57 kilograms). Mark's workouts enabled him to earn 93.5 health points and Linda's allowed her to earn 98.8, close to our optimal weekly recommended goal of 100.

OTHER AEROBIC EXERCISE CHOICES: THE PROS AND CONS

Table 4.5 provides information on how to calculate health points for other aerobic activities. To vary your routine, you may want to try some of these other forms of exercise. When doing so, keep in mind that these other forms of aerobic exercise require skill, are influenced by external factors such as the weather or terrain, or have not been adequately researched. Thus, although this table is extremely useful,

Mark

Date	Activity	Time	Distance/ work load	Health points	Notes
M	Walk	20 min	1.4 miles	13.8	Walking felt good.
	Schwinn Air-Dyne	20 min	2.0 WL	11.2	
T	Walk	30 min	2 miles	22.7	Walked farther today. A little tired, but okay.
W	Walk	15 min	1.1 miles	10.9	Blood-glucose level fluctuated a bit. Okay now.
	Schwinn Air-Dyne	25 min	1.8 WL	11.5	
F	Walk	20 min	1.4 miles	13.8	Good workout.
	Cycle (legs)	20 min	80 watts	9.6	
				93.5	**Total: Week** 20

Linda

Date	Activity	Time	Distance/ work load	Health points	Notes
M	Aerobics	40 min	13 RPE	21.2	No problems.
T	Walk	22-1/2 min	1.5 miles	16	Got a little light-headed.
	Schwinn Air-Dyne	15 min	1.3 WL	7.2	
W	Aerobics	45 min	12 RPE	23.9	Tough workout.
F	Walk	30 min	2 miles	22.7	Great day for a walk!
S	Swim	30 min	11 RPE	7.8	I took it easy today.
				98.8	**Total: Week** 28

it isn't as precise as those for walking, jogging, and stationary cycling. To use this table you need to know how long you exercised and whether you exercised at a light (RPE < 12), moderate (RPE = 12 to 13), or heavy (RPE > 13) intensity.

The ideal aerobic exercise for you has three basic characteristics:

- It's pleasant. You're more likely to stick with an exercise you enjoy.
- It is practical and fits into your lifestyle. In short, it's something you can do conveniently year-round.
- It uses large muscle groups. The larger the muscle groups you exercise, the greater your body's oxygen uptake will be. In addition to the exercises I've already discussed, the following exercises—and many others—fulfill this criterion.

Swimming

This is an excellent aerobic activity because it uses both the upper and lower body muscles. And because it's a non-weight-bearing activity, the chances of a musculoskeletal injury are extremely low. Swimming is especially valuable for people with lower back problems, arthritis, retinopathy, or heat-regulation disorders.

If you're overweight, shedding pounds through exercise should be one of your goals. Unfortunately, swimming may not help you as much in this regard as some other forms of aerobic exercise.[2] Exactly why this is, is not known, but it may be because swimming causes less rise in body temperature than other aerobic activities.

Aqua-Aerobics

This is just what the name implies—aerobic exercises done in water. The advantages and disadvantages of this increasingly popular low-impact sport are similar to those for swimming. If you find the prospect of exercising in a swimming pool appealing, see Ken Cooper's book *Overcoming Hypertension* for detailed guidelines.[3]

Cross-Country Skiing

Ken Cooper rates this as the top aerobics activity because "you have more muscles involved than just the legs; and any time you get more muscles involved, you get more aerobic benefit."[1] And the heavy clothing you wear and the weighty equipment you must carry further enhance the aerobic effect (that is, your energy expenditure) over that of walking or jogging at similar speeds.

There are drawbacks, though. The total exertion is greatly affected by variations in skill, snow surface, terrain, temperature and weather conditions, and altitude. Also, it's difficult to take your pulse in the middle of this activity. One way around these barriers is to use mechanical cross-country skiing devices, which some of our patients enjoy. They not only enable you to burn calories efficiently but also provide a low-impact activity that's unlikely to cause musculoskeletal or retinal problems.

Stair Climbing

These popular machines always seem to be in use at health clubs. They simulate the act of climbing flights of stairs, enabling you to work the large muscles in your back, buttocks, and legs and expend lots of energy quickly. Because stair climbing is strenuous and may cause a rapid rise in heart rate and blood pressure, it's generally not an appropriate activity for people with diabetic complications. Nor is it a good way for beginners to start an exercise program. If the idea of stair climbing appeals to you, wait until you've been working out for at least 8 weeks before adding it to your exercise regimen.[4]

People with knee problems should probably find another way to get an aerobic workout; stair climbing places stress on the knee joint that is thought to be equivalent to lifting four to six times your body weight. Needless to say, it's likely to aggravate existing problems in that area.[4]

Rope Skipping

This is a practical, enjoyable, and easily accessible aerobic activity. But it's not a popular choice, because it's relatively strenuous and may result in excessively high heart rates. Even at that, for a given heart rate, the energy expenditure is not as high as that for some other strenuous aerobic exercises, such as jogging. And it exposes you to the risk of musculoskeletal injuries—a significant drawback. Also, those of you with retinal problems should probably avoid this high-impact activity.

Aerobic Dance

Aerobic dancing involves steady, rhythmic movements done to the beat of relatively fast music, usually rock. Recently, benches that range in height from 6 to 12 inches (15 to 30 centimeters) have been introduced into aerobic dance workouts to increase the exercise intensity while reducing the impact and risk of injury. Linda Stone, and others like her with diabetes who enjoy aerobic dance, have improved their fitness via these "bench aerobics" workouts. Unfortunately, I cannot recommend aerobic dance for anyone with cardiac, vascular, or neurological diabetes complications unless the class is especially designed for them (and, frankly, I don't know of many). Aerobic dancing is very strenuous and will probably cause such people to exceed their training heart rate limit.

Circuit Resistance Training

This is a combination of aerobics and strength training. Typically an exerciser would use a series of resistance-training machines and move from one to another with very short rest periods—usually 15 to 30 seconds—in between. Performed correctly, circuit training improves the cardiovascular system, builds and tones muscles, and burns calories during one carefully constructed workout.

Sounds great, doesn't it? I didn't want to dismiss this exercise out of hand, so I reviewed the medical literature and we did our own study of its possible rehabilitation benefits.[5] Here's the catch: The primary benefit is enhancement of muscular strength, not energy expenditure. Thus, I do not recommend it for people with diabetes unless it's performed in conjunction with other forms of aerobic exercise.

It's best that people with cardiac, vascular, and neurological complications avoid circuit resistance training unless they have appropriate professional supervision and guidance from a doctor, nurse, or exercise physiologist with experience in prescribing exercise for people with chronic medical conditions. Even then, retinopathy patients may be placing themselves at undue risk because of the excessive rise in blood pressure that often occurs.

Recreational Sports

People who have no complications from their diabetes can participate in just about any exercise or sport. But people with chronic diabetes complications should be aware that once activities turn competitive, the risk of cardiovascular complications goes up. If you engage in recreational sports, you may have to modify the rules to minimize the competitive aspects and thus keep your heart rate within your designated limits. When performed in such a way, recreational sports can be, and often are, a valuable component of a diabetes rehabilitation exercise program.

Although I have not included sample introductory programs for each of these alternative exercise choices, it should be easy to use the walking and stationary cycling programs at the end of chapter 3 as a blueprint from which to formulate your own. For example, an introductory swimming program might be as follows:

Week	Duration per session	Frequency per week
1	7.5 minutes	3-5 times
2	10 minutes	3-5 times
3	12.5 minutes	3-5 times
4	15 minutes	3-5 times
5	17.5 minutes	3-5 times
6	20 minutes	3-5 times
7	25 minutes	3-5 times
8	30 minutes	3-5 times
9 and onward	It's time to start earning those 50 to 100 health points a week. Keep your exercise time at 30 minutes per session and gradually increase your swimming speed until you exceed 60% of your maximal heart rate (if you are not doing so yet). If this does not result in the desired weekly energy expenditure using the Other Aerobic Activities chart (Table 4.5, p. 79), do one or more of the following: Try exercising within the upper range of your target heart rate zone, exercise more frequently, or increase the duration of each exercise session.	

When using this swimming program (as with any aerobic exercise), start at a comfortable intensity. During the initial weeks, do not exceed 75% of your maximal heart rate and an RPE of 13. Also, be sure to warm up and cool down for at least five minutes each. You can do this by swimming slower or doing other activities in the water.

THE FOUR-LETTER WORD
YOU MUST NOT UTTER

That word is *quit*.

You've probably noticed I keep pushing the notion of *regular* exercise—not sporadic exercise, not fair-weather exercise, but the kind of persistent exercise you engage in almost daily because it's a habit, like brushing your teeth. There's a reason. When you exercise, your body and its organ systems are exposed to potent physiological stimuli. If you exercise regularly at an appropriate intensity and duration, these stimuli will result in specific adaptations that both enhance your ability to exercise and improve your health. In other words, you'll receive all the benefits of a physically active lifestyle that I outlined in chapter 2.

But these benefits can't be stored for a rainy day. They're reversible. All it takes to set this backtracking in motion is abstinence. If you stop training or reduce your physical activity below your required level, your body's systems soon readjust to this diminished amount of physiological stimuli. The result: Those hard-won, exercise-related gains, which you worked so long and hard to achieve, are lost.

This *reversibility concept* is best summed up by a landmark study of 16,936 Harvard University alumni by Ralph S. Paffenbarger, Jr., and his colleagues.[6] In this study, many former college athletes had become inactive adults. Consequently, they were in worse shape—and at greater risk for cardiovascular disease—than their contemporaries who had not participated in college sports but who had started exercising later in life. Researchers do not know how long it takes after you stop training before all the health benefits of exercise are lost. We do know that, even after many months of training, the resultant increase in insulin sensitivity is substantially diminished after only 2 or 3 days of inactivity. We also know that fitness declines rapidly during the first 12 to 21 days of inactivity, and the fitness benefits of regular exercise are almost totally lost after about 2 or 3 months.[7]

In view of this, it's imperative that you stick with your exercise program once you get started. Regrettably, this is easier said than done. Several studies on exercise compliance have shown that half or more of all patients drop out of their exercise programs within 6 months and that the critical dropout period is the first 3 months or so. You need motivators to get you through this critical time. The following suggestions will keep you huffing and puffing even when you'd rather be home in bed or watching television.

- *Make sure you fully understand the costs of not exercising versus the benefits of exercising.*

- *Start exercising slowly and progress gradually.*

- *Choose a form of exercise that's convenient as well as enjoyable.* If you constantly score below a "4" for enjoyment rating on

Exercise dropout rate

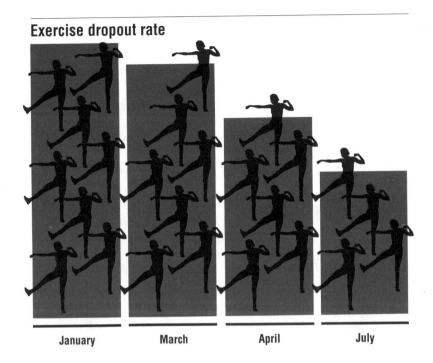

January	March	April	July

the exercise training log (pages 47-49), your exercise program needs to be modified.

• *Find a role model*—a friend, relative, or acquaintance who leads a physically active life. Find out why that person loves exercise so much.

• *Learn from your past exercise experiences.* Try to figure out where you went wrong previously.

• *Obtain as much support for your exercise program as possible.* Enlist the company—or, at the very least, the moral support—of those closest to you.

• *Bring your body to your place of exercise, even if your mind is temporarily on strike.* Special occasions, such as holidays or vacations, are no excuse.

• *Finally, remember that exercise is forever.* Physical activity is a lifelong pursuit.

Don't be an exercise dropout. I urge you to do everything in your power to stick with your exercise program, especially during the crucial initial months. Once you've passed the 6-month mark and tasted some of the tantalizing benefits of an active lifestyle, I think there's less and less chance you'll ever revert to unhealthy inactivity.

Table 4.1
Walking Health Points Chart

Time (min:sec)	Distance (miles)	Health points	Time (min:sec)	Distance (miles)	Health points
5:00	Under 0.10	0.8	7:30	Under 0.15	1.3
	0.10-0.14	1.0		0.15-0.19	1.5
	0.15-0.19	1.2		0.20-0.24	1.7
	0.20-0.24	1.4		0.25-0.29	1.9
	0.25-0.29	1.6		0.30-0.34	2.1
	0.30-0.33	1.8		0.35-0.39	2.3
	Over 0.33	*		0.40-0.44	2.5
				0.45-0.49	2.7
				Over 0.49	*
10:00	Under 0.20	1.7	12:30	Under 0.20	1.9
	0.20-0.24	1.8		0.20-0.29	2.3
	0.25-0.29	2.0		0.30-0.39	2.7
	0.30-0.34	2.2		0.40-0.49	3.1
	0.35-0.39	2.4		0.50-0.59	3.5
	0.40-0.44	2.6		0.60-0.69	3.9
	0.45-0.49	2.8		0.70-0.79	4.3
	0.50-0.54	3.0		0.80-0.83	4.7
	0.55-0.59	3.2		Over 0.83	*
	0.60-0.66	3.6			
	Over 0.66	*			
15:00	Under 0.30	2.5	17:30	Under 0.30	2.8
	0.30-0.39	2.9		0.30-0.49	3.5
	0.40-0.49	3.3		0.50-0.69	4.3
	0.50-0.59	3.7		0.70-0.89	5.1
	0.60-0.69	4.1		0.90-1.09	5.9
	0.70-0.79	4.5		1.10-1.16	6.7
	0.80-0.89	4.9		Over 1.16	*
	0.90-0.99	5.3			
	Over 0.99	*			
20:00	Under 0.40	3.4	22:30	Under 0.40	3.6
	0.40-0.59	4.1		0.40-0.59	4.4
	0.60-0.79	4.9		0.60-0.79	5.2
	0.80-0.99	5.7		0.80-0.99	6.0
	1.00-1.19	6.5		1.00-1.19	6.8
	1.20-1.33	7.3		1.20-1.39	7.6
	Over 1.33	*		1.40-1.49	8.4
				Over 1.49	*
25:00	Under 0.50	4.2	27:30	Under 0.50	4.5
	0.50-0.69	5.0		0.50-0.69	5.2
	0.70-0.89	5.8		0.70-0.89	6.0
	0.90-1.09	6.6		0.90-1.09	6.8

Time (min:sec)	Distance (miles)	Health points	Time (min:sec)	Distance (miles)	Health points
25:00 (Cont.)			27:30 (Cont.)		
	1.10-1.29	7.4		1.10-1.29	7.6
	1.30-1.49	8.2		1.30-1.49	8.4
	1.50-1.66	9.0		1.50-1.69	9.2
	Over 1.66	*		1.70-1.83	10.0
				Over 1.83	*
30:00	Under 0.50	4.6	35:00	Under 0.75	6.1
	0.50-0.74	5.6		0.75-0.99	7.0
	0.75-0.99	6.6		1.00-1.24	8.0
	1.00-1.24	7.6		1.25-1.49	9.0
	1.25-1.49	8.6		1.50-1.74	10.0
	1.50-1.74	9.6		1.75-1.99	11.0
	1.75-1.99	10.6		2.00-2.24	12.0
	Over 1.99	*		2.25-2.33	13.0
				Over 2.33	*
40:00	Under 1.00	7.5	45:00	Under 1.00	7.9
	1.00-1.24	8.5		1.00-1.49	9.9
	1.25-1.49	9.5		1.50-1.99	11.9
	1.50-1.74	10.5		2.00-2.49	13.9
	1.75-1.99	11.5		2.50-2.99	15.9
	2.00-2.24	12.5		Over 2.99	*
	2.25-2.49	13.5			
	2.50-2.66	14.5			
	Over 2.66	*			
50:00	Under 1.00	8.4	55:00	Under 1.00	8.8
	1.00-1.49	10.3		1.00-1.49	10.8
	1.50-1.99	12.4		1.50-1.99	12.8
	2.00-2.49	14.4		2.00-2.49	14.8
	2.50-2.99	16.4		2.50-2.99	16.8
	3.00-3.33	18.4		3.00-3.49	18.8
	Over 3.33	*		3.50-3.66	20.8
				Over 3.66	*
60:00	Under 1.00	9.3			
	1.00-1.49	11.2			
	1.50-1.99	13.2			
	2.00-2.49	15.2			
	2.50-2.99	17.2			
	3.00-3.49	19.2			
	3.50-3.99	21.2			
	Over 3.99	*			

*Use the Jogging Health Points Chart (Table 4.2).

Table 4.2
Jogging Health Points Chart

Time (min:sec)	Distance (miles)	Health points	Time (min:sec)	Distance (miles)	Health points
5:00	Under 0.40	3.6	7:30	Under 0.50	4.7
	0.40-0.49	4.4		0.50-0.59	5.4
	0.50-0.59	5.2		0.60-0.69	6.2
	0.60-0.69	6.0		0.70-0.79	7.0
	Over 0.69	6.8		0.80-0.89	7.8
				0.90-0.99	8.6
				1.00-1.09	9.4
				Over 1.09	10.2
10:00	Under 0.80	7.3	12:30	Under 1.00	9.2
	0.80-0.89	8.0		1.00-1.19	10.7
	0.90-0.99	8.8		1.20-1.39	12.3
	1.00-1.09	9.6		1.40-1.59	13.9
	1.10-1.19	10.4		1.60-1.79	15.5
	1.20-1.29	11.2		Over 1.79	17.1
	1.30-1.39	12.0			
	1.40-1.49	12.8			
	Over 1.49	13.6			
15:00	Under 1.20	10.9	17:30	Under 1.40	12.8
	1.20-1.39	12.5		1.40-1.59	14.3
	1.40-1.59	14.1		1.60-1.79	15.9
	1.60-1.79	15.7		1.80-1.99	17.5
	1.80-1.99	17.3		2.00-2.19	19.1
	2.00-2.19	18.9		2.20-2.39	20.7
	Over 2.19	20.5		2.40-2.59	22.4
				Over 2.59	24.0
20:00	Under 1.50	13.8	22:30	Under 1.75	16.0
	1.50-1.74	15.7		1.75-1.99	18.0
	1.75-1.99	17.7		2.00-2.24	20.0
	2.00-2.24	19.7		2.25-2.49	22.0
	2.25-2.49	21.7		2.50-2.74	24.0
	2.50-2.74	23.7		2.75-2.99	26.0
	2.75-2.99	25.7		3.00-3.24	28.0
	Over 2.99	27.7		Over 3.24	30.0
25:00	Under 2.00	18.2	27:30	Under 2.00	18.5
	2.00-2.24	20.2		2.00-2.24	20.4
	2.25-2.49	22.2		2.25-2.49	22.4
	2.50-2.74	24.2		2.50-2.74	24.4
	2.75-2.99	26.2		2.75-2.99	26.4
	3.00-3.24	28.2		3.00-3.24	28.4
	3.25-3.49	30.2		3.25-3.49	30.4
	3.50-3.74	32.2		3.50-3.74	32.5

Time (min:sec)	Distance (miles)	Health points	Time (min:sec)	Distance (miles)	Health points
25:00 (Cont.)			27:30 (Cont.)		
	Over 3.74	34.2		3.75-3.99	34.5
				Over 3.99	36.5
30:00	Under 2.50	22.7	35:00	Under 2.75	25.1
	2.50-2.74	24.6		2.75-2.99	27.0
	2.75-2.99	26.6		3.00-3.24	29.1
	3.00-3.24	28.6		3.25-3.49	31.1
	3.25-3.49	30.6		3.50-3.74	33.1
	3.50-3.74	32.6		3.75-3.99	35.1
	3.75-3.99	34.6		4.00-4.24	37.1
	4.00-4.24	36.6		4.25-4.49	39.1
	Over 4.24	38.6		4.50-4.74	41.1
				4.75-4.99	43.1
				Over 4.99	45.1
40:00	Under 3.00	27.6	45:00	Under 3.50	32.0
	3.00-3.49	31.5		3.50-3.99	35.9
	3.50-3.99	35.5		4.00-4.49	40.0
	4.00-4.49	39.5		4.50-4.99	44.0
	4.50-4.99	43.5		5.00-5.49	48.0
	5.00-5.49	47.5		5.50-5.99	52.0
	5.50-5.99	51.6		6.00-6.49	56.0
	Over 5.99	55.6		Over 6.49	60.0
50:00	Under 4.00	36.5	55:00	Under 4.50	40.9
	4.00-4.49	40.4		4.50-4.99	44.8
	4.50-4.99	44.4		5.00-5.49	48.9
	5.00-5.49	48.4		5.50-5.99	52.9
	5.50-5.99	52.4		6.00-6.49	56.9
	6.00-6.49	56.4		6.50-6.99	60.9
	6.50-6.99	60.4		7.00-7.49	64.9
	7.00-7.49	64.5		7.50-7.99	68.9
	Over 7.49	68.5		Over 7.99	72.9
60:00	Under 4.50	41.3			
	4.50-4.99	45.3			
	5.00-5.49	49.3			
	5.50-5.99	53.3			
	6.00-6.49	57.3			
	6.50-6.99	61.3			
	7.00-7.49	65.3			
	7.50-7.99	69.3			
	8.00-8.49	73.4			
	8.50-8.99	77.4			
	Over 8.99	81.4			

Table 4.3
Stationary Cycling (Legs Only) Health Points Chart

	Health points per minute							
Work rate (watts)	Under 100 lb	100 to 124 lb	125 to 149 lb	150 to 174 lb	175 to 199 lb	200 to 224 lb	225 to 249 lb	Over 249 lb
Under 25	0.34	0.28	0.24	0.22	0.20	0.18	0.17	0.16
25-49	0.54	0.44	0.36	0.32	0.28	0.26	0.24	0.22
50-74	0.76	0.60	0.50	0.42	0.38	0.34	0.32	0.30
75-99	0.98	0.76	0.62	0.54	0.48	0.42	0.38	0.36
100-124	1.20	0.92	0.76	0.64	0.56	0.50	0.46	0.42
125-149	1.42	1.10	0.90	0.76	0.66	0.58	0.54	0.48
150-174	1.64	1.26	1.02	0.86	0.76	0.68	0.60	0.56
175-199	1.86	1.42	1.16	0.98	0.84	0.76	0.68	0.62
200-224	2.08	1.58	1.28	1.08	0.94	0.84	0.76	0.68
225-249	2.30	1.76	1.42	1.20	1.04	0.92	0.82	0.76
Over 249	2.52	1.92	1.56	1.30	1.14	1.00	0.90	0.82

Table 4.4
Schwinn Air-Dyne Health Points Chart

	Health points per minute							
Work load	Under 100 lb	100 to 124 lb	125 to 149 lb	150 to 174 lb	175 to 199 lb	200 to 224 lb	225 to 249 lb	Over 249 lb
Under 0.5	0.34	0.28	0.24	0.22	0.20	0.18	0.17	0.16
0.5-0.9	0.52	0.40	0.34	0.30	0.26	0.24	0.22	0.21
1.0-1.4	0.74	0.56	0.48	0.40	0.36	0.32	0.30	0.28
1.5-1.9	0.96	0.74	0.60	0.52	0.46	0.42	0.38	0.34
2.0-2.4	1.18	0.90	0.74	0.62	0.56	0.50	0.44	0.42
2.5-2.9	1.40	1.06	0.86	0.74	0.64	0.58	0.52	0.48
3.0-3.4	1.62	1.22	1.00	0.84	0.74	0.66	0.60	0.54
3.5-3.9	1.84	1.40	1.14	0.96	0.84	0.74	0.66	0.62
4.0-4.4	2.06	1.56	1.26	1.06	0.92	0.82	0.74	0.68
4.5-4.9	2.28	1.72	1.40	1.18	1.02	0.90	0.82	0.74
Over 4.9	2.50	1.88	1.52	1.28	1.12	0.98	0.88	0.80

Table 4.5
Other Aerobic Activities

| Activity | Health points per minute | | |
| | Intensity* | | |
	Light	Moderate	Heavy
Aerobic dancing	0.35	0.53	0.79
Alpine skiing	0.35	0.53	0.70
Aqua-aerobics	0.35	0.53	0.79
Arm-cycle ergometry	0.22	0.35	0.61
Backpacking	0.53	0.70	0.88
(5% slope, 44 lb or 20 kg)			
4.0 mph (6.4 kph)	0.70		
4.5 mph (7.2 kph)	0.84		
5.0 mph (8.0 kph)	1.02		
6.0 mph (9.6 kph)	1.15		
7.0 mph (11.2 kph)	1.36		
Badminton	0.26	0.53	0.79
Ballet	0.44	0.53	0.70
Ballroom dancing	0.26	0.35	0.44
Baseball	0.26	0.35	0.44
Basketball	0.53	0.70	0.96
Bicycling	0.26	0.61	0.88
6.3 mph (10 kph)	0.42		
9.4 mph (15 kph)	0.52		
12.5 mph (20 kph)	0.62		
15.6 mph (25 kph)	0.74		
18.8 mph (30 kph)	0.86		
Canoeing	0.26	0.35	0.53
Catch (ball)	0.26	0.35	0.44
Circuit resistance training	0.26	0.44	0.61
Cricket	0.26	0.35	0.44
Cross-country skiing	0.44	0.79	1.14
2.5 mph (4 kph)	0.48		
3.8 mph (6 kph)	0.67		
5.0 mph (8 kph)	0.87		
6.3 mph (10 kph)	1.07		
7.5 mph (12 kph)	1.25		
8.8 mph (14 kph)	1.44		
Exercise classes	0.35	0.53	0.79
Fencing	0.44	0.61	0.88
Field hockey	0.53	0.70	0.88
Figure skating	0.35	0.53	0.88

(Cont.)

Table 4.5
(Continued)

| Activity | Health points per minute | | |
| | Intensity* | | |
	Light	Moderate	Heavy
Football (American)		0.44	0.53	0.61
Football (touch)		0.44	0.53	0.70
Golf				
Carrying clubs	0.45			
Pulling cart	0.35			
Riding cart	0.22			
Gymnastics		0.44	0.61	0.88
Handball (4-wall)		0.53	0.70	0.96
Hiking		0.26	0.53	0.70
Home calisthenics		0.26	0.44	0.70
Hunting		0.26	0.44	0.61
Ice hockey		0.53	0.70	0.88
Judo		0.53	0.70	1.05
Karate		0.44	0.70	1.05
Kayaking		0.53	0.70	0.96
7.8 mph (12.5 kph)	0.68			
9.4 mph (15.0 kph)	0.96			
Lacrosse		0.53	0.70	0.88
Modern dancing		0.44	0.53	0.70
Mountaineering		0.61	0.70	0.88
Orienteering		0.70	0.88	1.05
Racquetball		0.53	0.79	1.05
Rebounding		0.31	0.44	0.53
Rollerskating		0.44	0.57	0.70
Rope skipping		0.61	0.88	1.05
66 per min	0.86			
84 per min	0.92			
100 per min	0.96			
120 per min	1.00			
125 per min	1.02			
130 per min	1.03			
135 per min	1.05			
145 per min	1.06			
Rowing		0.61	0.88	1.14
2.5 mph (4 kph)	0.48			
5.0 mph (8 kph)	0.90			
7.5 mph (12 kph)	1.18			
10.0 mph (16 kph)	1.44			

Activity	Health points per minute		
	Intensity*		
	Light	Moderate	Heavy
Rowing (Cont.)			
12.5 mph (20 kph)	1.67		
Rugby	0.53	0.70	0.96
Scuba diving	0.35	0.44	0.53
Sculling	0.35	0.53	0.88
Skateboarding	0.44	0.57	0.70
Skating (ice)	0.35	0.61	1.14
11.3 mph (18 kph)	0.35		
15.6 mph (25 kph)	0.42		
17.5 mph (28 kph)	0.81		
20.0 mph (32 kph)	0.95		
22.5 mph (36 kph)	1.33		
Snorkeling	0.35	0.44	0.53
Soccer	0.44	0.61	0.96
Softball	0.26	0.35	0.44
Squash	0.53	0.79	1.05
Stair climbing	0.35	0.61	0.96
Swimming (beach)	0.18	0.26	0.35
Swimming (pool)	0.26	0.44	0.79
1.3 mph (2 kph)	0.38		
1.6 mph (2.5 kph)	0.60		
1.9 mph (3.0 kph)	0.78		
2.2 mph (3.5 kph)	1.01		
2.5 mph (4.0 kph)	1.19		
Synchronized swimming	0.35	0.53	0.70
Table tennis	0.26	0.44	0.70
Tennis	0.35	0.53	0.88
Volleyball	0.44	0.53	0.70
Walking up stairs	0.35	0.53	0.70
Water polo	0.53	0.70	0.96
Wrestling	0.53	0.79	1.05

*Light intensity results in minimal perspiration and only a slight increase in breathing above normal (RPE of less than 12). Moderate intensity results in definite perspiration and above normal breathing (RPE of 12-13). Heavy intensity corresponds to heavy perspiration and breathing (RPE of more than 13). These values are adapted from an expert committee report of the Canada Fitness Survey - source M. Jette et al., Clinical Cardiology, 13 (1990): 555-565.

Chapter 4
Prescription

❏ If you're a novice exerciser, consider using one of my beginning programs. And let your doctor help you adapt it to suit your medical condition.

❏ Use our Health Points System to gain optimal health benefits with minimal risk.

❏ When using the Health Points System, adjust your frequency, intensity, and duration of exercise to earn 50 to 100 points each week.

❏ Do not attempt to earn your quota of health points in fewer than three workouts—on at least 3 separate days—each week.

❏ Keep your goals realistic and modify them continually as your condition permits.

❏ If your condition is such that you cannot attain the desired weekly health points, don't become discouraged. If you perform some type of aerobic exercise for a minimum of 15 minutes at least 3 days a week, you'll gain important health benefits.

❏ Be proud of whatever progress you are able to make.

❏ Do everything in your power to keep from becoming an exercise dropout, especially during the crucial initial months.

Chapter 5

How to Prevent a Blood-Sugar Emergency

E xercise is never completely risk-free, even for people without chronic diseases. But when you've got diabetes, you have the added concern that injudicious exertion can precipitate a blood-sugar emergency.

Type II diabetes patients who are unmedicated—that is, not on oral hypoglycemic agents or insulin—should be able to exercise without worrying about being caught off-guard by a blood-sugar emergency. However, the same can't be said for those with Type II on medication or those with Type I.

Exercising when your blood-glucose levels are poorly controlled is risky. When a healthy person exercises, the pancreas decreases its insulin secretion while other glands increase their secretion of "counterregulatory" hormones. This combination increases glucose release from the liver into the bloodstream. However, because some insulin is present in the blood (and only small amounts are needed during exercise), the active muscles can take up more glucose for energy production. Thus, blood-glucose levels remain steady (see Figure 5.1a).

However, when you exercise with a severe insulin deficiency, you're flirting with *hyperglycemia*—a high-blood-sugar emergency—because there is a greater than normal increase in counterregulatory hormone secretion. This, together with insulin deficiency, causes the liver to

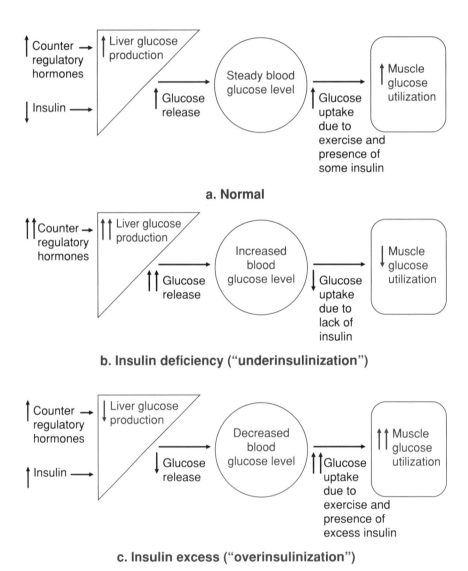

Figure 5.1   How insulin deficiency and insulin excess affect blood-glucose levels during exercise.

release excessive quantities of glucose into the bloodstream. And due to a lack of insulin in the blood, the active muscles cannot take up this excess glucose, resulting in increased blood-glucose levels (see Figure 5.1b).

In contrast, anyone on insulin who exercises when there is too much of this medication in the bloodstream risks *hypo*glycemia—a low-blood-sugar emergency—because the excess insulin causes the liver to release too little glucose into the bloodstream while also enabling the active muscles to take up large amounts of glucose from the blood for energy production. This causes a net fall in blood-glucose levels (see Figure 5.1c). Because oral hypoglycemic agents foster the body's production of and/or response to insulin, people with Type II diabetes who take them are also candidates for low-blood-sugar problems.

Table 5.1 describes the three major kinds of blood-sugar emergencies.

SELF-MONITORING: WHAT EVERY EXERCISER ON DIABETES MEDICATION MUST LEARN TO DO

Monitoring your own blood glucose is one of the best ways to prevent a blood-sugar emergency. The beauty of self-monitoring is that it can be done anywhere, anytime—even on an exercise track. It's a vital information tool for persons who want to maintain daily control over their condition. For exercisers with diabetes—especially those taking insulin or oral hypoglycemic agents—self-monitoring is indispensable. *You must learn how to do it.*

To monitor your blood glucose, you can test either your urine or your blood.

Urine Testing

Urine glucose testing was once the mainstay of diabetes self-monitoring. You place some urine on a chemically impregnated strip or tablet, and if your blood-glucose level is so high (usually exceeding 180 mg/dl) that excess glucose is spilling over into your urine, the strip changes color to indicate you're in the hyperglycemia danger zone. The problem is that a urine glucose test can only tell you when you're already in trouble, not when you're simply approaching it. Even worse, it only

Table 5.1
Three Kinds of Blood-Sugar Emergencies

Condition	Description
Hypoglycemia	*Hypo* means low. *Glycemia* means blood-glucose level. A dangerously low blood-sugar level is the most common problem for people with Type I diabetes, and for those with Type II who are on insulin therapy or take oral hypoglycemic agents.
Hyperglycemia with ketoacidosis	*Hyper* means high. Hence, this condition is a dangerously high blood-sugar level accompanied by an excessive accumulation of *ketones* in the bloodstream (which in turn increases blood acidity, triggering *acidosis*). Untreated hyperglycemia and ketoacidosis can lead to a coma. People with Type I diabetes are prone to this condition, but generally people with Type II need worry about it only during periods of severe physical or emotional distress. Early warning symptoms are drowsiness, incessant urination, and intense thirst.
Hyperglycemic coma of the nonketotic, hyperosmolar type	People with Type II diabetes have a tendency toward this type of coma, which is caused by unchecked high blood-glucose levels (*hyperglycemic*) where the blood shows no signs of ketoacidosis (*nonketotic*). The result is dehydration, triggering more concentrated blood (*hyperosmolar*), which can lead to coma. Early warning symptoms are drowsiness, incessant urination, and intense thirst.

indicates when your blood glucose level is too high; it's almost useless in detecting *hypo*glycemia.

Another type of urine test, which detects ketones, is more useful. It's performed in a similar way to urine glucose testing. A urine ketone test is the only practical way you can test for excessive amounts of ketones in your blood. The combination of high concentrations of glucose and ketones in the blood is serious because it indicates a dangerous insulin deficiency.

Whenever your blood-glucose level is above 240 mg/dl or the glucose in your urine exceeds 1%, do a ketone test—especially if you have Type I diabetes. If ketones are present, call your health-care team immediately. The combination of high glucose in the blood and excessive ketones in the urine indicates a potentially dangerous condition known as *ketoacidosis*. Untreated ketoacidosis can lead to a coma. Patients with Type I diabetes are prone to this condition. Those with Type II should worry about it only during periods of severe physical or emotional distress.

Blood-Glucose Self-Monitoring

This is a relatively new innovation. All medicated diabetes patients must test their blood glucose to prevent exercise-induced hypoglycemia. Thanks to recent technological advances, self-monitoring of blood glucose is easy. You can assess your blood sugar quickly and accurately with any of several small, portable monitoring devices. Most are the size of a pocket calculator; some are as small as a pen.[1]

Here's how they work. You prick your finger and place a drop of blood on a chemically impregnated strip. The strip changes color according to your blood's glucose content, and the monitoring device reads it and tells you your blood-sugar content in mg/dl. There's also a less accurate, visual method of reading the strip yourself, called color estimation. You match the strip with a color reference chart that gives blood-glucose values in mg/dl.

It's important to self-monitor during exercise. How you do it depends on the type of exercise. For instance, if you exercise on a stationary cycle, you can easily continue pedaling while monitoring your blood-sugar level. If you're walking, running, or swimming, you'll have to stop to do it. Most blood-glucose meters give results within 30 seconds to 2 minutes.

If you don't know how to self-monitor, ask a member of your health-care team to show you how. Teaching you this valuable procedure is one of your health-care team's responsibilities.

Your doctor, who knows your medical condition and lifestyle, can tell you when and how often to self-monitor. He or she can also figure out the ideal blood-glucose values you should aim for at various times of day. By self-monitoring, you'll know if you're meeting them. For an estimate of what's generally considered acceptable and ideal, see Table 5.2. To avoid hypoglycemia, people who take insulin should aim for values somewhat above the lower limits in this table.

SELF-MONITORING AND EXERCISE TIPS

For people who take insulin or oral hypoglycemic agents, self-monitoring is the key to preventing hypoglycemia during and after workouts.

Table 5.2
Appropriate Blood-Glucose Levels

Time of day	Acceptable level	Ideal level
Fasting, including before breakfast	70-130 mg/dl	70-100 mg/dl
Before meals other than breakfast	70-140 mg/dl	70-110 mg/dl
1 hour after meals	Below 200 mg/dl	Below 160 mg/dl
2 hours after meals	Below 150 mg/dl	Below 120 mg/dl
3 a.m.	Above 70 mg/dl	Above 70 mg/dl

Note. Adapted from D.W. Foster, "Diabetes Mellitus," in E. Braunwald et al. (Eds.), *Harrison's Principles of Internal Medicine*, 11th edition. New York: McGraw-Hill, 1987. Also, L.P. Krall and R.S. Beaser, *Joslin Diabetes Manual*, 12th Ed. Philadelphia: Lea and Febiger, 1989.

(As I'll explain in chapter 6, the risk for hypoglycemia is actually greatest *after* rather than *during* exercise.) By self-monitoring your blood glucose, you can determine whether you need to reduce an insulin dosage, eat extra carbohydrates, or both. To help you control your diabetes, in this section I share some tips about self-monitoring and exercise.

**HYPOGLYCEMIA PREVENTION TIP FOR PATIENTS
WITH TYPE II DIABETES ON SULFONYLUREA DRUGS**

Self-monitor your blood-glucose levels both before and immediately after exertion.

Some people with Type II diabetes cannot control their chronic high blood sugar with correct nutrition and exercise, try as they might. Their doctors may prescribe oral hypoglycemic agents. These medications lower blood-glucose levels, often by stimulating the pancreatic insulin secretions and reducing other cells' resistance to taking in glucose. Sulfonylurea drugs are currently the only U.S. Food and Drug Administration-approved oral hypoglycemic agents.

Taking sulfonylurea drugs places you at higher risk for developing the opposite problem—*hypo*glycemia, or low blood sugar—when you exercise. Ironically, this is particularly true if your blood-glucose levels are usually well controlled.

DRUG ALERT FOR PEOPLE WITH TYPE II DIABETES

Ask your doctor if any medications you're taking put you at greater risk for a hypoglycemic attack during exercise. If you're about to stop taking a drug, also ask what risks this poses and for how long.

The best antidote to a hypoglycemic reaction is to self-monitor your blood sugar both immediately before and after exercise, and sometimes during. This not only minimizes your risk for hypoglycemia but also gives you vital feedback on how your body responds to exercise. Then you can apply what you learn to future exercise sessions.

Here's the rule of thumb: *If your workout will last for longer than 60 minutes, self-monitor your blood glucose at least every 30 to 60 minutes.* After you've been doing this for a while and feel confident you've achieved a stable balance between exercise and medication intake, you'll be able to self-monitor less frequently.

Self-monitoring guidelines for people on sulfonylurea drugs

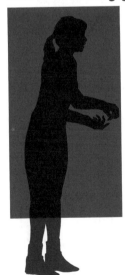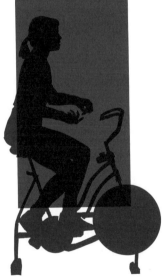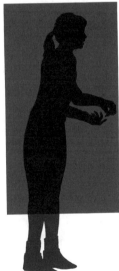

Self-monitor before exercise

Self-monitor during exercise

Self-monitor after exercise

HYPOGLYCEMIA PREVENTION TIP FOR EXERCISERS ON INSULIN

Self-monitor your blood-glucose levels before, during, and after exercise.

The primary concern for persons on insulin, whether your diabetes is Type I or II, is hypoglycemia. Until you know how your body reacts to exercise, it's a good idea to self-monitor your blood sugar before and after exercise, and every 15 to 30 minutes during exercise. Once you know what's normal for you, you can self-monitor less often—before and after exercise, and every 20 to 60 minutes during workouts lasting longer than an hour.

Use the readings you take during exercise to screen for signs of hypoglycemia. Remember to consider your blood-glucose values in relation to each other. Watch for large changes from one reading to the next. For example, two consecutive readings of 100 mg/dl is as stable as you can get, whereas a value of 140 mg/dl followed by a value of 100 is a warning sign of possible impending hypoglycemia.

The magnitude of the decline in your blood sugar is related to your pre-exercise value. The higher your pre-exercise blood-glucose level, the larger the decline you can expect. Conversely, the lower your pre-exercise blood-glucose level, the smaller the probable drop.[2]

If you're taking insulin (or an oral hypoglycemic agent, for that matter) and your pre-exercise blood-glucose level is below 100 mg/dl, eat a snack 15 to 20 minutes before starting exercise. This precaution will reduce your risk for hypoglycemia.

HYPOGLYCEMIA PREVENTION TIP FOR EXERCISERS ON INSULIN

Ask your doctor to help you coordinate your insulin regimen with your daily exercise schedule. Then fine-tune the insulin dosages in accordance with your self-monitored blood-glucose levels.

To prevent hypoglycemia, many people taking insulin—whether their diabetes is Type I or II—need to reduce their insulin dose before exercise. The amount by which to reduce it depends on several factors. (See Appendix C, "Hypoglycemia Prevention Checklist.") In truth, so many variables are involved that I doubt it will ever be possible (or, for that matter, appropriate) to provide specific guidelines for all patients at all times. So consider the guidelines in this book a mere starting point for tailoring and individualizing your insulin regimen with the help of your health-care team.

In general, these are the three most important factors affecting your insulin dose:

- Your blood-glucose level prior to insulin injection. The higher your blood sugar, the less you'll need to reduce your dose.
- The intensity and duration of your exercise. Generally, the greater the intensity and duration, the more you'll have to reduce your dose. The exception is very-high-intensity exercise of short duration (sprint-type exercise), which is more likely to cause *hyper-* than *hypo*glycemia.
- The time lag between insulin injection and exercise. The greater the time interval, the less you'll need to reduce your dose.

Self-monitoring your blood glucose before and after exercise is the starting point for fine-tuning your insulin dosages. I have found that Type I diabetes patients who participate in a regular, long-term exercise program are able to decrease their total daily dose of insulin by as much as 15% to 20%. If your blood-glucose levels are always very low (that is, below 80 mg/dl) before a prolonged, one-hour-plus exercise session, you definitely must talk to your doctor about adjusting your insulin dosages to accommodate exercise.

If you take insulin, ask your doctor this question: *Which insulin dose, if any, do I need to reduce before a scheduled exercise session?* In all likelihood, your physician will advise you to reduce the insulin dose that will be acting in your body during your exercise workout. Usually only insulin injections taken on the day of exercise need to be reduced. Table 5.3 will give you an idea as to when regular, NPH, and ultralente insulin injections exert their greatest effects. If you intend to work out when one of these injections is most active, you may need to reduce the dosage.

The following is a sample chart for recording the information your doctor gives you about modifying your insulin dosages before exercise:

My Exercise Timetable and Insulin Therapy		
Insulin regimen (type of insulin & injection schedule)	Daily exercise time(s) (especially when prolonged exercise is planned)	Insulin dose that should be reduced before my scheduled exercise session(s)

Table 5.3
When Injected Insulin
Exerts Its Greatest Blood-Glucose-Lowering Effect

Type of insulin	Time injected	Period of greatest blood-glucose-lowering activity
Regular	Before a meal	Between that meal and either the next one or the bedtime snack (if insulin is taken before supper). Action usually starts 0.5-1 hour after injection and reaches a peak 2-4 hours after injection.
NPH	Before breakfast	Between lunch and supper. Action usually starts 3-4 hours after injection and reaches a peak 10-16 hours after injection.
NPH	Before supper or before bedtime	Overnight.
Ultralente	Before breakfast or before supper, or half of the dose at each time	Mostly overnight because regular insulin overrides its effect during the day. Action usually starts 6-8 hours after injection and reaches a peak 14-20 hours after injection.

Note. Adapted from M.B. Davidson. "How to Get the Most Out of Insulin Therapy." *Clinical Diabetes* 8 (1990): 65-73.

Pro golfer Sherri Turner credits the advice and support of her health-care team as being the reason that, about 5 years ago, she was finally able to gain control of her blood-sugar levels—some 13 years after her Type I diabetes was first diagnosed when she was 15.[3] And it's possible that getting her blood glucose under better control helped her capture the Ladies Professional Golf Association Championship in 1988.

Looking back, Sherri regrets the years of worrying about having a blood-sugar emergency on the greens. When she was a teenager, her family doctor put her on one insulin injection a day and let it go at that. She was not taught how to self-monitor her blood glucose and adjust the insulin dosages accordingly.

"Diabetes was real scary," Sherri said. "I didn't know it was something I could control. I'd catch myself on the golf course having low blood sugar. I'd start feeling kind of weak and perspiring and I'd get a little shaky."

In 1986, she decided to learn more about her diabetes. She saw a team of specialists—a physician who was an insulin expert, a nutritionist, and a psychologist—at the Texas Institute of Diabetes in Houston. They switched her to human insulin (which she admits took some getting used to) and introduced her to self-monitoring, a wonderful concept that's freed up Sherri's life. But Sherri says regulating her insulin dosages wasn't easy at first because, as she soon discovered, her body's needs were different when she was on the road playing versus when she stayed home doing paperwork. Today, Sherri has one insulin dosage schedule for days at home, another for noncompetitive practice days, and two possible regimens during tournaments, depending on when the competition is scheduled.

HYPERGLYCEMIA EMERGENCY PREVENTION TIP
FOR EVERYONE WITH DIABETES—
BUT ESPECIALLY THOSE WITH TYPE I

If your pre-exercise blood-glucose level is higher than 240 mg/dl, check your urine for ketones before exercising. If ketones are present, or if your blood-glucose level is higher than 300 mg/dl, don't exercise.

Exercising when your blood-glucose level is excessively high may worsen your blood-sugar control and increase your risk for ketoacidosis and coma. If you're taking insulin and you have both high blood sugar and ketones in your urine, consider giving yourself an injection. Then postpone exercise until ketones are no longer present in your urine.

(It's also a good idea to contact your health-care team and let them know about it.)

Another scenario may require a quite different response. If your blood-glucose level is between 240 and 300 mg/dl and no ketones are present in your urine, exercise may actually be beneficial because it tends to lower your blood-glucose count. However, a count above 300 mg/dl, even if no ketones are in your urine, is a serious matter. Don't exercise if your blood-glucose count is above 300 mg/dl. Gain control of your blood sugar through diet and insulin injections or oral hypoglycemic agents before you continue your exercise program.

EATING AND EXERCISE: SOME PRACTICAL ANSWERS

When it comes to preventing low-blood-sugar emergencies during or after exercise, correct nutrition is of paramount importance. I encourage our exercising diabetes patients to ask questions and to let us know when they're confused. Here is a roundup of my patients' most common queries about achieving the right balance between exercise, diet, and diabetes medication.

Q: *How important is it to have a dietitian working with me on meal planning?*

A: Ideally, you want a health-care team of experienced professionals helping you to learn about and control your diabetes through eating and exercise. A registered dietitian is an important member of that team. Initially, a dietitian will counsel you about the basic aspects of good nutrition, which, let's face it, constitute survival skills for people with diabetes. Then, the dietitian will hone in on your individual case, working out a meal pattern to suit your special lifestyle and exercise needs.

Q: *I take insulin, which makes planning drug injections, meals, and exercise more difficult because they all affect my blood-sugar metabolism and glucose levels. To prevent hypoglycemia, what should my eating and exercise schedule be?*

A: I recommend to our Type I and Type II diabetes patients on insulin that they implement a twofold strategy that mimics what happens in the bodies of healthy people when they exercise (see Figure 5.1). First, reduce your circulating insulin levels before exercise. Second, consume additional carbohydrate only when your exercise session lasts longer than 45 minutes, your blood-glucose level is low, or you start to experience hypoglycemic symptoms (see chapter 6).

One way to do this is to exercise after eating a regularly scheduled meal or snack. Exercising 1 to 3 hours after meals or snacks, when your blood-glucose level is likely to be above 100 mg/dl, may be ideal because the exertion may actually improve your blood-glucose reaction to the food you've just eaten. However, exercising at that time may still be a threat unless you've also reduced the insulin dose that's active during your workout. From the standpoint of preventing hypoglycemia, it's more important to exercise when circulating insulin levels are lower than when blood-glucose levels are higher.

If you experience exercise-induced hypoglycemia, try lengthening the interval between exercise and your insulin injections. This ensures you'll be exerting yourself when your circulating insulin levels are lower.[4] A Mayo Clinic study even suggests that before breakfast may be the best time for some insulin-dependent diabetes patients to work out to avoid hypoglycemia.[5] Not only are blood-insulin levels likely to be low then, but in some patients blood-glucose levels tend to rise between 6 and 9 a.m., aptly termed the dawn phenomenon.

Another phenomenon, known as the Somogyi phenomenon, could also account for a regular early-morning rise in blood sugar.[6] Named after the physician who first described it more than 50 years ago, the Somogyi phenomenon is a rebound reaction in which an excessive fall in blood glucose due to too much insulin medication (see Figure 5.1) during the night stimulates the release of counterregulatory hormones, which, in turn, causes a *hyper*glycemic reaction. It's likely you're experiencing the Somogyi phenomenon if you have daily fluctuations between hypo- and hyperglycemia; you have ketones, but *not* sugar, in your urine in the morning; or you awaken in the morning with symptoms suggestive of nighttime hypoglycemia. To see if you are, in fact, experiencing nighttime hypoglycemia, measure your blood glucose between 2 and 4 a.m.

If your early-morning rise in blood sugar is due to the Somogyi phenomenon, you need to reduce your evening insulin dose. In this situation, before-breakfast exercise could actually heighten your risk for hypoglycemia.

Q: *Could you discuss the interrelationship between dietary factors, insulin and oral hypoglycemic agent dosage reductions, and my workout's expected intensity and duration?*

A: Generally, if all of the following four conditions are present, I recommend that you eat no additional carbohydrate either before or during exercise:

- Your pre-exercise blood-glucose levels are above 100 mg/dl.
- The exercise session will be only moderate in intensity and will last for 45 minutes or less.

- If you're taking insulin, the session will take place no sooner than 1 hour after an insulin injection.
- The insulin or oral hypoglycemic agent dosage will be in an appropriate amount, more than likely reduced from the usual dosage.

I advise that rather than automatically eating carbohydrate beforehand, moderately active exercisers with diabetes should self-monitor their blood glucose before and after their workouts and then eat carbohydrate only if it's clearly needed to prevent hypoglycemia. Of course, for exercise lasting longer than 45 minutes, patients often find that they must eat extra carbohydrate before and during exercise to prevent a hypoglycemic reaction.

It's difficult to give a hard-and-fast rule about how much carbohydrate to eat before and during exercise to stave off hypoglycemia. But there are equations that can help determine this. Those equations enabled me to offer the rough guidelines given on pages 95 to 97.[7]

I've known of instances where patients followed the guidelines to the letter and their blood-glucose levels still dropped to between 60 and 100 mg/dl during workouts. If this happens to you, consume 10 to 15 grams of carbohydrate, even if you are not scheduled to do so. Then, as you continue your exercise session, measure your blood glucose at least every 20 to 30 minutes. If necessary, eat even more carbohydrate than scheduled. Continually watch for symptoms of hypoglycemia. If you experience any, or if your blood-glucose level ever falls below 60 mg/dl, follow the guidelines I outline in chapter 6.

Q: *What can a person with Type II diabetes who takes oral hypoglycemic agents do to achieve that stable balance between exercise, carbohydrate consumption, and medication?*

A: You've got three choices: increase carbohydrate intake before, after, and, if necessary, during exercise; reduce your drug dosage; or both.

I recommend first trying to reduce your drug dosage. To a certain extent, finding the right dosage is a matter of trial and error. If you'll be exercising for longer than 30 minutes within 1 to 2 hours after taking your medication, it may be prudent to reduce or completely eliminate the dose. Even if the interval between drug ingestion and exercise is longer—say, you take a dose in the morning and exercise in the late afternoon—you may find an adjustment is necessary.

But the trial-and-error method won't work unless you exercise at a consistent pace and duration each session so that the same metabolic conditions apply. Diabetes patients have to be more regimented than other people about their exercise schedule. In diabetes patients, spontaneity and abrupt changes in the pattern of their exertion may cause trouble, particularly if self-monitoring of blood glucose is not done.

TAILORING YOUR DIET AND INSULIN REGIMEN TO YOUR EXERCISE INTENSITY AND DURATION

This advice is geared to diabetes patients exercising at an intensity of 60% to 75% of their maximal heart rate, which roughly corresponds to 12 to 13 on the Borg Perceived Exertion Scale shown in chapter 3. These guidelines are to be used as a starting point only. I encourage you to fine-tune your diet and insulin regimen further based on your self-monitored blood-glucose results and in consultation with your health-care team.

Exercise duration: Less than 15 minutes

- *Pre-exercise insulin dosage adjustment:* It's unlikely you'll need to make any change.
- *Diet:* If your pre-exercise blood-glucose level is below 80 mg/dl, eat 10 to 15 grams of extra carbohydrate before you exercise.
- *After exercise:* Self-monitor your blood glucose. If it's below 80 mg/dl and it's not time for a scheduled meal or snack, eat 10 to 15 grams of carbohydrate, more if necessary.

Exercise duration: 15-30 minutes

- *Pre-exercise insulin dosage adjustment:* If you intend to exercise within 3 hours after a short-acting insulin injection (or bolus for insulin pump users*), reduce the amount of that injection by 10%.
- *Diet:* If your pre-exercise blood-glucose level is below 100 mg/dl, eat 10 to 15 grams of extra carbohydrate before you exercise.
- *After exercise:* Self-monitor your blood glucose. If it's below 80 mg/dl and it's not time for a scheduled meal or snack, eat 10 to 15 grams of carbohydrate, more if necessary.
- *Postexercise insulin dosage adjustment:* Adjust according to your self-monitored blood-glucose results.

(Continued)

TAILORING YOUR DIET AND INSULIN REGIMEN TO EXERCISE (Continued)

Exercise duration: 31-45 minutes

- *Pre-exercise insulin dosage adjustment:* If you'll be exercising within 3 hours after a short-acting insulin injection (or bolus for insulin pump users*), reduce the amount of that injection by 20%.
- *Diet:* If your pre-exercise blood-glucose level is below 100 mg/dl, eat 20 to 30 grams of extra carbohydrate before you exercise.
- *After exercise:* Self-monitor your blood glucose. If it's below 80 mg/dl and it's not time for a scheduled meal or snack, eat 10 to 15 grams of carbohydrate, more if necessary.
- *Postexercise insulin dosage adjustment:* Adjust according to your self-monitored blood-glucose results.

Exercise duration: 46-60 minutes

- *Pre-exercise insulin dosage adjustment:* If you'll be exercising within 3 hours after a short-acting insulin injection (or bolus for insulin pump users*), reduce the amount of that injection by 30%.
- *Diet:* If your pre-exercise blood-glucose level is below 100 mg/dl, eat 10 to 15 grams of extra carbohydrate before you exercise.
- *During exercise:* Slow down or stop briefly at 15- or 20-minute intervals and eat 10-15 grams of carbohydrate. (Even if you stop to drink or eat, continue to move your legs in place.)
- *After exercise:* Self-monitor your blood glucose. If it's below 80 mg/dl and it's not time for a scheduled meal or snack, eat 10 to 15 grams of carbohydrate, more if necessary.
- *Postexercise insulin dosage adjustment:* Adjust according to your self-monitored blood-glucose results.

Exercise duration: More than 1 hour

- *Pre-exercise insulin dosage adjustment:* If you'll be exercising after a short- or longer-acting insulin injection (or bolus for insulin pump users*) is at work in your body, reduce the amount of the injection by 10% of your total insulin dose for the whole day that you'll be exercising on. Do whatever the arithmetic says, unless the reduction in a short-acting insulin dosage is less than 30%. Under such circumstances, reduce the amount of that injection by 30%.

For example, at one stage Linda Stone's total daily insulin dose was 34 units—6 regular and 18 NPH before breakfast and 2 regular and 8 NPH before dinner. When she exercised for more than an hour, she reduced each of her regular and/or NPH insulins acting at the time of exercise by about 3 units. The arithmetic—34 units × 10% = 3.4—rounded off to 3 units. When Linda exercised in the morning after breakfast, her pre-breakfast insulin doses were 3 regular (6 − 3) and 18 NPH; when she exercised in the afternoon, her pre-breakfast insulin doses were 6 regular and 15 NPH (18 − 3); and when she exercised in both the morning and afternoon, her pre-breakfast insulin doses were 3 regular (6 − 3) and 15 NPH (18 − 3).

Work with your health-care team to decide which insulin doses need reducing during prolonged exercise.

- *Diet:* Even if your pre-exercise blood-glucose level is above 100 mg/dl, eat 20 to 30 grams of carbohydrate before you begin exertion.
- *During exercise:* Slow down or stop briefly at 15- or 20-minute intervals and eat 10 to 15 grams of carbohydrate.
- *Self-monitoring during exercise:* Self-monitor your blood glucose at least every hour without fail.
- *After exercise:* Self-monitor your blood glucose. If it's below 80 mg/dl and it's not time for a scheduled meal or snack, eat 10 to 15 grams of carbohydrate, more if necessary.
- *Postexercise insulin dosage adjustment:* Adjust according to your self-monitored blood-glucose results.

---

*Exercisers on insulin-pump therapy have to grapple with a decision unique to their situation: Do I reduce my basal insulin infusion rate or the insulin bolus given before a meal? Or do I instead stop the pump completely during exercise?

Generally, a reduction in the basal infusion rate (by approximately 50%) during exercise and a reduction in the before-meal insulin bolus preceding your exercise session are sufficient measures to prevent hypoglycemia during any workout that's no longer than 45 to 60 minutes. The bolus should be reduced in accordance with the above recommendations for short-acting insulin. For longer workouts, insulin-pump patients should do three things: reduce the before-meal insulin bolus; turn off the pump completely during exercise; and reduce the basal infusion rate by 25% to 50% for several hours after the workout ends, depending on their postexercise blood-glucose levels.[8]

Balancing exercise, carbohydrate consumption, and medication

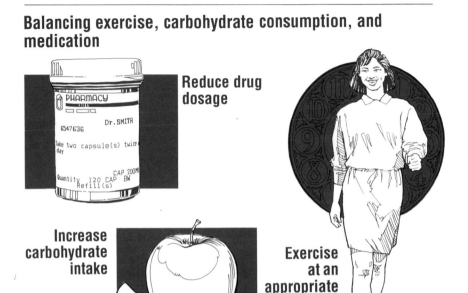

Reduce drug dosage

Increase carbohydrate intake

Exercise at an appropriate time

Despite reducing your drug dosage or even omitting it completely on the days your workout lasts longer than 30 minutes, you may find that your pre-exercise blood-glucose level is still below 100 mg/dl. If this happens, increase your carbohydrate intake by 20 to 30 grams before exercise and, if necessary, during exercise (follow the dietary recommendations given on pages 95 to 97 for persons receiving insulin therapy). In addition, talk to your doctor about the possibility of reducing your drug dosage substantially on a long-term basis (not just before exercise)—or even going off it completely.

I also recommend that you follow the dietary recommendations for persons receiving insulin therapy if you take a sulfonylurea drug, have a pre-exercise blood-glucose value below 180 mg/dl, and intend to exercise for more than 60 minutes.

Let's take another set of circumstances: Your pre-exercise blood-glucose level is about right, but your blood-glucose level during exercise falls to between 60 and 100 mg/dl. What do you do? Immediately eat or drink 10 to 15 grams of carbohydrate, even if you're not scheduled to do so. Also, monitor your blood glucose at 20- to 30-minute intervals during the rest of your workout. You may have to consume more carbohydrate than scheduled to get your levels back on a more even keel.

This is very important: If you ever develop symptoms of hypoglycemia or, even in the absence of symptoms, should your blood-sugar level fall below 60 mg/dl, consider it a serious emergency and follow the hypoglycemia prevention guidelines in chapter 6.

Q: *I control my Type II diabetes through a careful diet and do not take medication. What special things do I have to do to accommodate exercise?*

A: You're lucky. You shouldn't have to concern yourself with the guidelines I have outlined because you're not at significant risk for exercise-induced hypoglycemia. But if the glucose in your urine exceeds 1%, test your urine for ketones. They are unlikely to be present, but if they are, notify your health-care team and do not exercise until your diabetes is under better control. If you exercise anyway, your blood-glucose control is likely to worsen rather than improve. The same applies if your blood-glucose levels are ever above 300 mg/dl: Even in the absence of urinary ketones, don't exercise.

One final word of advice: If you intend to exercise longer than 90 minutes, you may need to eat carbohydrate before and during exercise to prevent hypoglycemia, just as a savvy exerciser without diabetes should. How much? Eat about 10 to 15 grams of carbohydrate before you start your workout. During your workout, slow down or stop briefly at 15- or 20-minute intervals and eat another 10 to 15 grams.

Q: *What snacks are ideal for consumption during prolonged exercise sessions?*

A: What type of carbohydrate should exercising diabetes patients eat or drink? That's a controversial topic. There's no clear consensus among the experts about which is better in exercise situations—rapidly absorbed simple carbohydrates or snacks containing complex carbohydrates. Frankly, I've found that both types of foods have pros and cons, so it's a toss-up.

Although simple carbohydrates, such as those in most commercial sports drinks, may effectively prevent hypoglycemia when consumed before and during a workout, they can raise a diabetes patient's blood sugar steeply. And because they're absorbed rapidly into the blood, their effect on blood glucose is sometimes not a sustained one. So to prevent hypoglycemia, they must be consumed frequently during long workouts, about every 15 to 20 minutes.

In contrast, complex carbohydrate foods, such as the starches and raw fruits listed in the chart that follows, are absorbed more slowly. They don't need to be consumed as frequently during exercise, and they're less likely to boost blood glucose excessively. But eating solid food during exercise may cause stomach discomfort; some people's digestive systems just can't take it. Also, some research suggests that eating snacks, rather than drinking sports beverages containing only 5% to 10% carbohydrate, can interfere with the body's fluid absorption and thereby increase the risk for dehydration.[9] On the latter point, more research is needed.[10]

Most professional and competitive athletes consume sports drinks rather than snacks during exercise. Experiment with both approaches and decide what's best for you. Some of my patients prefer a combination. They eat a complex carbohydrate snack before prolonged exercise and drink a sports beverage during exercise. The chart I give our exercising diabetes patients is shown in the box on page 101.

Q: *I'm a serious athlete who happens to have diabetes. Can I do carbohydrate loading before an important competition?*

A: This practice—which involves gorging on complex carbohydrates such as bread and pasta for about 3 days before a marathon race or some other prolonged (more than 90 minutes) and intense athletic competition—has been studied by numerous biochemical researchers. It's been proved that this practice does increase muscle carbohydrate stores and exercise performance. However, none of these studies involved people with diabetes, and most diabetes experts advise their patients against it. Frankly, I've found that for most people with Type I diabetes, the practice is more likely to impair rather than enhance performance.

To do carbohydrate loading, a person with Type I diabetes would need to make special adjustments to insulin dosages. And it's probably too dangerous for most patients to experiment with this practice to figure out those dosages. What's dangerous about it? Excessively high blood-glucose levels that may result from carbohydrate loading can cause dehydration, among other things. And dehydration during exercise increases your risk for heatstroke.

Despite my warning, if you're determined to try carbohydrate loading before a big athletic event, ask your health-care team to assist you. For more information on this and related issues, I suggest serious athletes with diabetes consult an excellent book called *Diabetes: Actively Staying Healthy* by Marion Franz and Jane Norstrom.[11] They may also want to join the International Diabetic Athletes Association (the address is IDAA, 1931 E. Rovey Ave., Phoenix, AZ 85016). This is an outstanding organization of people with diabetes who participate in sports of all kinds. In addition to publishing a newsletter and holding an annual meeting, the organization serves as a rapidly expanding worldwide networking system.

SNACKS SUITABLE
FOR EXERCISE-RELATED CONSUMPTION

Starches (about 15 grams carbohydrate and 80 calories each)

8 animal crackers
1/2 bagel (1 oz.)
2 crisp bread
 sticks, each 4 in.
 × 1/2 in.
 (2/3 oz)

1/2 English muffin
3 graham crackers,
 each 2-1/2 in.
pretzels (3/4 oz)

4 rye crisp, each
 2 in. × 3-1/2 in.
6 saltine crackers
2-4 wafers of no-
 fat-added, whole
 wheat crackers,
 such as Finn,
 Kavli, Wasa
 (3/4 oz)

Fruits (about 15 grams carbohydrate and 60 calories each)

Raw fruit	Dried fruit	Fruit juice
1 apple, 2 in. across	4 apple rings	1/2 cup apple juice or cider
1/2 banana, 9 in. long	7 apricot halves	1/3 cup cranberry juice cocktail
1/2 medium grapefruit	2-1/2 medium dates	1/2 cup grapefruit juice
15 small grapes	1-1/2 figs	1/3 cup grape juice
1 nectarine, 2-1/2 in. across	3 medium prunes	1/2 cup orange juice
1 orange, 2-1/2 in. across	2 tablespoons raisins	1/2 cup pineapple juice
1 small pear		
2 plums, each 2 in. across		

Low-fat milk products (about 12 grams carbohydrate and 90 calories each)

1 cup skim milk
1 cup 1/2%-fat milk

1 cup 1%-fat milk
8 oz plain nonfat yogurt

Chapter 5
Prescription

❒ Learn how to self-monitor your urine for glucose and ketones.

❒ Learn how to self-monitor your blood glucose, especially if you're taking insulin or oral hypoglycemic agents.

❒ If you are taking insulin or oral hypoglycemic agents, self-monitor your blood glucose before and after your workouts. Also do so during prolonged exercise.

❒ If your pre-exercise blood-glucose level is more than 300 mg/dl, or if it's more than 240 mg/dl and ketones are present in your urine, don't exercise.

❒ Tailor your diet and insulin regimen to your expected exercise intensity and duration.

❒ Ask your doctor to help you coordinate your insulin regimen with your daily exercise schedule. You may need to reduce your usual insulin dosage before workouts.

Chapter 6

Staying Out of the Danger Zone: Essential Exercise Guidelines for People With Diabetes

Fortunately, prescribing exercise as medical therapy for diabetes patients no longer has to be guesswork. Today, well-informed physicians can prescribe exercise just as they would a drug. However, as is the case with drugs, certain precautions are in order to make sure your exercise regimen is both safe and effective.

SEVEN SAFE-EXERCISE GUIDELINES

In this chapter, I discuss the special hazards associated with exercise for people with Types I and II diabetes. And I offer additional advice on how to minimize your risk of having an exercise-related, blood-glucose emergency.

EXERCISE SAFETY GUIDELINE 1:

Obtain a detailed medical evaluation before you begin your exercise program and at regular intervals thereafter.

The American Diabetes Association recommends that anyone with diabetes, regardless of age, have a thorough medical exam before starting an exercise program.[1] In Appendix B, you'll find a checklist of what that exam should include—and guidelines for how frequently you should have follow-up checkups.

For some diabetes patients, the risks of exercise may outweigh the benefits, although very few can't exercise at all. The contraindications to exercise are outlined in the following checklist. Over time, some of the conditions can be corrected and thus eliminated as roadblocks to exercise. Others cannot.

✓ Do *NOT* Exercise if Your Physician Indicates You Have Any ✓ of These Conditions

Diabetes patients with one or more of these conditions should not exercise until therapy or the passage of time controls or corrects their problems. Ask your doctor if you have any of the following:

_____ A blood-glucose level above 300 mg/dl

_____ A blood-glucose level above 240 mg/dl and ketones in the urine

_____ Untreated high-risk proliferative retinopathy

_____ Recent significant bleeding in the eye (if you have retinopathy)

_____ Kidney failure that is not under adequate control

_____ Severe autonomic neuropathy that could cause a dangerous fall in systolic blood pressure during exercise

_____ Unstable angina pectoris

_____ Recent significant change in resting ECG that has not been adequately investigated and managed

_____ A recent embolism

_____ Thrombophlebitis or an intracardiac thrombus

_____ Active or suspected myocarditis or pericarditis

_____ Acute or inadequately controlled heart failure

_____ Moderate to severe aortic stenosis

_____ Clinically significant hypertrophic obstructive cardiomyopathy

_____ Suspected or known aneurysm (cardiac or vascular) that your physician thinks may be worsened by exercise

_____ Uncontrolled atrial or ventricular arrhythmias that are considered to be clinically significant

_____ Resting heart rate greater than 100 beats per minute

_____ Third-degree heart block

_____ Uncontrolled hypertension with resting systolic blood pressure above 180 mmHg or diastolic blood pressure above 105 mmHg

_____ Recent fall in systolic blood pressure of more than 20 mmHg that was not caused by medication

_____ Uncontrolled metabolic disease, such as thyrotoxicosis or myxedema

_____ Acute infection or fever

_____ Chronic infectious disease—such as mononucleosis, hepatitis, or AIDS—that your doctor thinks may be worsened by exercise

_____ Significant electrolyte disturbances

_____ Neuromuscular, musculoskeletal, or rheumatoid disorders that may be made worse by exercise, in your physician's opinion

_____ Major emotional distress (psychosis)

_____ Any other condition known to be a contraindication to exercise

---

You may have thought all chronic diabetes complications, mild though some may be, would preclude any possibility of exercise for you. Not so. Most complications put exercise off-limits only if you don't have access to an exercise facility where there's medical supervision. If you have any of the following conditions, you should begin exercising in a medically-supervised program: cardiac problems, peripheral vascular disease, preproliferative or proliferative retinopathy, autonomic neuropathy, kidney problems, minimally controlled blood-glucose levels, or difficulty in preventing hypoglycemia during exertion. If no significant problems develop in the first 12 weeks of regular exercise, you may or may not need to continue the on-site medical supervision. It depends on how confident you are about going it alone and what your doctor says.

You may have noticed that pregnancy was not included in the list of contraindications to exercise. Studies of pregnant women with Type I diabetes have shown that they may be able to participate in a strictly supervised exercise program without adverse effects.[2] But their insulin requirements tend to vacillate, sometimes on a daily basis, and many experts believe the risks of exercise may outweigh the benefits. For pregnant women who have Type I or II diabetes and who also have other significant medical conditions (or obstetrical complications including being at risk for premature labor), it may be best not to exercise at all. Discuss your particular circumstances with your doctor.

The 2nd International Workshop-Conference on Gestational Diabetes Mellitus recommended (and other authorities agree) that women with uncomplicated Type II diabetes and those with gestational diabetes who had an active lifestyle before their pregnancy may continue a program of moderate exercise, provided it's closely supervised.[3] (Gestational diabetes is brought on by pregnancy and usually abates after the pregnancy ends.) A supervised program may also benefit pregnant women with uncomplicated Type II diabetes or gestational diabetes who were previously sedentary.

Here's some special advice for pregnant women: Always monitor your blood glucose before and after exercise. Be especially careful to adjust your diet—and, if applicable, insulin dosages and timing—in order to prevent hypoglycemia. Pregnancy places all women with diabetes at a much higher risk for hypoglycemia during the first 4-1/2 months of their term. Ken and Millie Cooper's book *The New Aerobics for Women*[4] gives specific, in-depth exercise guidelines for pregnant women. In general, a pregnant woman who has diabetes should exercise at the lower end of her training target heart rate zone and should follow the standard guidelines for all pregnant women.

EXERCISE SAFETY GUIDELINE 2:

Know the warning signs of an impending cardiac complication.

The information I've given you about exercise safety is not meant to scare you away. Exercise is a more normal state for the human body than indolence, and most people with diabetes, even those taking insulin, can exercise with confidence.

It comes down to this: You're probably far more likely to die from the deleterious effects of sedentary living than you are to die suddenly during exercise. But it's still prudent to keep your risk as low as reasonably possible. One of the best ways to boost your benefit-to-risk ratio is to remember this axiom:

Although death during exercise is always unexpected, it's seldom unheralded.

In other words, you'll often have some warning of cardiac complicatons. The box on page 108 lists the bodily signs that indicate possible heart problems. If you experience any of them before, during, or just after your exercise sessions, discuss it with your doctor before continuing with your workout program.

EXERCISE SAFETY GUIDELINE 3:

Put safety at the top of your exercise priority list by following proper exercise protocol.

When it comes to exercise, there's a right way and a wrong way to do it, a safe way and a dangerous way. Everyone who exercises should follow general safety guidelines. (For a detailed description of these general guidelines, see one of these books from the Cooper Clinic: *Running Without Fear*,[5] *The Aerobics Program for Total Well-Being*,[6] or *The New Aerobics for Women*.[4]) The following guidelines are especially relevant for exercisers with diabetes:

• *Warm up and cool down adequately—allow a minimum of 5 minutes for each.* Sufficient warm-up and cool-down are important for every exerciser because more than 70% of cardiac problems that surface during exercise do so either at the beginning or end of a session. Warm-up and cool-down are even more critical for people with autonomic neuropathy.

• *Don't exercise in adverse climatic conditions, particularly without taking adequate precautions.* Hyperthermia, an overheating of the body during exercise, not only impairs your ability to exercise

WARNING SIGNS OF HEART PROBLEMS

✓ *Pain or discomfort in your chest, abdomen, back, neck, jaw, or arms.* Such symptoms may be signs of an inadequate supply of blood and oxygen to your heart muscle due to potentially serious conditions such as atherosclerotic plaque buildup in your coronary arteries.

✓ *A nausea sensation during or after exercise.* This can result from a variety of causes, but it can also signify a cardiac abnormality.

✓ *Unaccustomed shortness of breath during exercise.* Any kind of aerobic exercise may make you huff and puff. This isn't what I'm referring to. But if you ordinarily walk 3 miles in 45 minutes with no breathlessness and one day you can't do it anymore, you should be alarmed.

✓ *Dizziness or fainting.* This could also be a sign of hypoglycemia. It can also occur in people without diabetes who don't follow proper exercise protocol and fail to cool down adequately. Stopping exercise suddenly could make anyone feel momentarily dizzy or even actually faint. The type of dizziness I'm concerned about occurs while you're exercising rather than on stopping. This is a more probable sign of a serious heart problem and warrants immediate medical consultation.

✓ *An irregular pulse, particularly when it's been regular in your past exercise sessions.* If you notice what appears to be extra heartbeats or skipped beats, notify your doctor. This might not mean anything of significance, but it could point to heart problems.

but also predisposes you to heatstroke, a potentially fatal condition. People with diabetes, particularly those with autonomic neuropathy, are especially prone to it.

Many symptoms of hyperthermia—headache, dizziness, confusion, stumbling, nausea, cramps, cessation of sweating, or excessive sweating—are also typical of both cardiac problems and hypoglycemia, making it somewhat difficult to distinguish between these reactions. To prevent hyperthermia, take these four preventive measures:

- If you're exercising outdoors, let weather conditions guide the amount and intensity of exercise you do on a given day. When heat and humidity are high, don't engage in strenuous exercise.

- Drink fluids while you're exercising, especially on hot days. Do this even if you're not thirsty. About 15 minutes before you begin your session, drink about 8 ounces (or 240 milliliters) of cold water (which is absorbed more quickly than lukewarm water). If your workout lasts longer than 30 minutes, take another 8-ounce drink at 15- to 20-minute intervals during exercise.
- When exercising in warm weather, wear clothing that promotes heat loss. Fabrics that "breathe," such as a mesh or fishnet T-shirt, are good choices.
- If you must exercise in the heat, sponge off the exposed parts of your body with cool water at regular intervals.

- *Take adequate precautions for cold-weather workouts.* Cold-weather exercise sessions pose challenges for people with diabetes, especially those who have peripheral neuropathy or heart disease. Be sure to wear gloves and a hooded sweatshirt or woolen cap to cover your head. Choose clothing that provides adequate insulation from the cold, but avoid fabrics that cause excessive buildup of sweat. Multiple layers of clothing are a good choice for cold-weather workouts. Also, use good judgment about exercising in the cold. Stay

Symptoms of hyperthermia

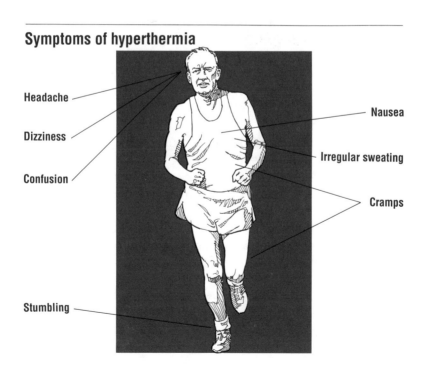

Headache

Dizziness

Confusion

Nausea

Irregular sweating

Cramps

Stumbling

indoors when the windchill index falls below 15 °F (–10 °C). If it's icy or slippery, don't exercise outdoors.

• *Pay special attention to proper foot care.* Diabetes patients are at great risk for foot problems. They are prone to peripheral vascular disease, which causes poor circulation to the feet, and to peripheral neuropathy, which decreases a person's ability to perceive pain and pressure and thus masks foot injuries. They also have problems with foot infections.

Proper foot care is crucial for anyone with diabetes who exercises because even minor infections and cuts in the feet can lead to a very severe infection called *gangrene*. Gangrene, as those of you familiar with old war movies know, can require amputation of the foot or leg below the knee. Lower-limb amputations are about 15 times more common in people with diabetes than in other people. In 1985 in the United States alone, more than 50,000 amputations were performed on diabetes patients. Proper foot care can reduce such alarming statistics. Several large American clinical centers have reduced the rate of amputations among diabetes patients by 44% to 85%, solely by implementing foot-care education programs.[7] The boxes on pages 110 and 111 list my recommendations for proper foot care.

FOOTCARE GUIDELINES
FOR PEOPLE WITH DIABETES WHO EXERCISE

• Be especially careful in selecting shoes. Buy shoes that are comfortable, fit correctly, and are specially designed for exercises you'll be doing.

• Before donning shoes, particularly before exercising, check for objects such as pebbles that could injure your feet.

• Wear socks that are smooth, not nubby, and *change them every day.* After a workout, immediately put on a clean, dry pair of socks. Sweaty socks increase your susceptibility for athlete's foot.

• Never exercise barefoot. Don't even walk around barefoot— not anywhere, but especially not in locker rooms, where you should not even shower barefoot. If you do, you risk contracting athlete's foot.

• Wash your feet in warm, soapy water every day, but *do not soak them in water.* Soaking softens the skin and increases your susceptibility to infection.

(Continued)

FOOTCARE GUIDELINES (Continued)

- *Never wash your feet in hot water or apply heat of any other kind to your feet.* For example, don't put hot water bottles, heating pads, or electric blankets on or around your feet. When checking the temperature of your bathwater, use your fingers or elbow, not your feet.
- Always dry your feet carefully, especially between your toes. Never allow your feet to remain continually moist. If necessary, apply powder daily to absorb excess moisture from the skin.
- But don't allow your feet to get too dry, either. If the skin on your feet becomes dry, apply a moisturizing lotion with lanolin every day until the dryness subsides. *Apply the lotion sparingly between your toes.*
- Inspect (or have a family member inspect) your feet daily, including between your toes. Look for scratches, cuts, blisters, ingrown toenails, corns, and calluses that may be present even though you feel no discomfort. Do this inspection whether or not you exercise that day. Have corns and calluses pared off routinely by your doctor or podiatrist; *do not do it yourself.* Most foot ulcers start under pressure areas, which such sites are.
- File rather than cut your toenails. File them straight across and diagonally at the corners. U-shaped nails predispose you to ingrown toenails.
- Report any signs of athlete's foot or infection immediately to your doctor. Even if your feet seem fine, ask to have your feet examined during every visit with your health-care team.

EXERCISE SAFETY GUIDELINE 4:

Memorize the symptoms of hypoglycemia.

Hypoglycemia is the major risk of exercise for diabetes patients who take insulin or oral hypoglycemic agents. Symptoms of moderate and severe hypoglycemia (see the box on page 112) are caused by an inadequate supply of glucose to the brain. When such a condition

---

WARNING SIGNS OF HYPOGLYCEMIA

Mild hypoglycemic reaction

✓ Trembling or shakiness
✓ Nervousness
✓ Rapid heart rate
✓ Palpitations
✓ Increased sweating
✓ Excessive hunger

Moderate hypoglycemic reaction

✓ Headache
✓ Irritability and other abrupt mood changes
✓ Impaired concentration and attentiveness
✓ Mental confusion
✓ Drowsiness

Severe hypoglycemic reaction

✓ Unresponsiveness
✓ Unconsciousness and coma
✓ Convulsions

---

is prolonged or happens repeatedly, you can sustain irreparable damage to your brain and nervous system. Mild hypoglycemic symptoms are more of a nuisance than anything else, but take them seriously. They result from the release of adrenaline-like hormones in the body's attempt to raise your blood-sugar level. Generally, you won't experience even mild symptoms until blood-glucose levels drop below 50 to 60 mg/dl.

These symptoms can vary considerably from one person to the next. Not only that, not all people with diabetes can depend on hypoglycemic symptoms to warn them of an impending low-blood-sugar emergency. For example, patients with autonomic neuropathy lose the ability to release adrenaline-like hormones in response to low blood sugar; they have a condition known as *hypoglycemic un-awareness*. They must monitor their blood sugar regularly during exercise, because that's the only way they'll know if they've got low-blood-sugar problems—until it's too late. People who take beta-blocker medications, which block the action of adrenaline-like hormones, are also at greater risk for hypoglycemic unawareness.

EXERCISE SAFETY GUIDELINE 5:

Know the six steps to take immediately *in the event of a hypoglycemia attack.*

Step 1. Don't hesitate to take action even if you're not entirely sure that it's hypoglycemia causing your symptoms. Hypoglycemia reactions come on suddenly and worsen quickly. If you wait too long and it is hypoglycemia, you soon won't be able to think clearly enough to get yourself out of your predicament. Worse yet, you could be unconscious.

Step 2. Stop exercising and, if at all possible, test your blood-glucose level to confirm that your problem is, indeed, hypoglycemia.

Step 3. Eat or drink 10 to 15 grams of simple carbohydrate or whatever quantity has proved to be effective previously. Always have some form of simple carbohydrate with you while exercising. Some suggestions are 4 to 6 ounces of orange or other fruit juice; 5 or 6 LifeSavers; 1 tablespoon of honey or Karo syrup; 4 teaspoons of sugar; 2 large or 5 small sugar cubes; 1 box (2 tablespoons) of raisins; 3 glucose tablets (available at any drugstore); 1/2 tube of Glutose (80-gram container); 1/2 tube of Insta-Glucose (31-gram container); or 1-1/2 packages of Monojel. Ice cream and chocolates might not do the job for you, because their high-fat content impedes the quick absorption of simple sugars into the bloodstream.

Step 4. Take at least a 10- or 15-minute rest to allow the carbohydrate to take effect. Before resuming exercise, retest your blood-glucose level. If it's below 100 mg/dl or you still don't feel right and suspect you haven't recovered completely, repeat the above steps.

Step 5. For the remainder of your exercise session, pay close attention to any signals you get from your body so that you can be sure the hypoglycemic reaction is truly over. Also, measure your blood-glucose level at least every 20 to 30 minutes during the remainder of your workout.

Step 6. If you don't have a meal scheduled right after exercise, at least eat a snack that contains complex carbohydrates.

If a severe hypoglycemic reaction can't be righted with carbohydrate ingested orally, you may need a subcutaneous glucagon injection or an intravenous injection of glucose. (Glucagon is a hormone that a healthy person's pancreas secretes to boost blood-glucose levels.) Intravenous glucose, injected directly into a vein, should be administered by a trained health-care professional. Glucagon, on the other hand, can be administered by a friend, relative, or exercise partner via the same method you use for insulin. However, it's up to you to have a supply of glucagon on hand. It's a good idea to coach your close friends and associates in injection techniques beforehand. You should also make those around you fully aware of what constitutes a hypoglycemic reaction.

It's smart to assume you may have a blood-sugar emergency one day, despite using the checklist in Appendix C for preventing hypoglycemia. Prepare for it by educating your family and friends about what to do. Show them where your carbohydrate snack foods are. Provide them with a list of emergency telephone numbers. Above all, carry adequate identification on you at all times that says you have diabetes, or wear a medical ID bracelet. I don't advise diabetes patients who take insulin or oral hypoglycemic agents to exercise alone, especially for sessions longer than an hour or so.

EXERCISE SAFETY GUIDELINE 6

Be aware that late-onset hypoglycemia can occur 4 or more hours after you've stopped exercising.

Most medicated diabetes patients are aware of their tendency to have low blood sugar during or right after exercise so they're careful to see it doesn't happen. The same people often don't realize that hypoglycemia remains a threat for much longer. Insulin sensitivity usually remains high for 24 to 48 hours after a person stops exercising. *It's now believed that late-onset hypoglycemia, which occurs up to 48 hours after a workout, is more common than hypoglycemia during or immediately after exercise.*[8] (The official definition of late-onset hypoglycemia is excessively low blood sugar occurring more than 4 hours after the end of exercise.)[8]

Preparing for a blood-sugar emergency

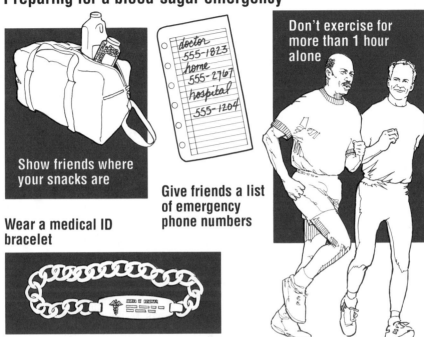

Show friends where your snacks are

Wear a medical ID bracelet

Give friends a list of emergency phone numbers

Don't exercise for more than 1 hour alone

You can guard against late-onset hypoglycemia by taking the following precautions:

Precaution 1. Be aware that hypoglycemia can strike up to 48 hours after exercise if you're being treated with insulin or oral hypoglycemic agents. Also, it's more prevalent among new exercisers or those who've just finished a particularly hard or long session.

Precaution 2. Use foresight. Adjust your insulin or oral hypoglycemic agent dosage before exercise and, if warranted, increase your food intake before and during exercise. (Consult the box beginning on page 95 in chapter 5.)

Precaution 3. After any exercise sessions longer than 45 minutes, keep monitoring your blood glucose at 2-hour intervals for 12 hours— or until bedtime. If warranted, reduce your insulin doses (mainly your regular insulin doses) or oral hypoglycemic agent doses during the remainder of the day and most especially at night. Over this time, if your blood-glucose level falls below 80 mg/dl, eat extra complex carbohydrates if a meal or snack is not scheduled. Before bedtime, a sandwich and glass of milk are good antidotes to overnight hypoglycemia.

Precaution 4. Monitor your blood glucose for 12 hours after exercise whenever you begin a new form of exercise or make a major change in intensity or duration—even if the workout is shorter than 45 minutes.

Precaution 5. Let your body get used to exercise gradually. Don't try to become fit in a week or two. Even for people without diabetes, going from little or no exercise to an obsession with working out is dangerous.

EXERCISE SAFETY GUIDELINE 7:

Don't believe the myth that injecting insulin into a part of the body that won't be active during exercise will prevent hypoglycemia.

At one time, even many diabetes experts believed that injecting insulin into a part of the body that would be nonactive during exercise— for example, switching from a thigh to an abdomen site before jogging—might substantially reduce the risk for hypoglycemia. This myth was based on the fact that the absorption of insulin from the subcutaneous tissue of an exercising body part is accelerated.

While the latter may be true, recent studies have shown that unless exercise is done immediately after an insulin injection, this measure is of little or no value.[9] And insulin is usually absorbed more rapidly from the abdomen than from the thigh or arm, so switching from these sites to the abdomen before exercise could increase your risk for hypoglycemia.

Changing your injection site to a nonexercising area such as your abdomen may reduce your risk for hypoglycemia if you begin exertion immediately after injecting insulin, but it is unlikely to help much if you wait more than 30 minutes. And this isn't a good idea for the reason I previously explained: *It's not smart to begin exercising until at least an hour after an insulin injection, no matter where the injection site.*

By following these exercise safety guidelines and self-monitoring blood-glucose levels, most people with diabetes can exercise safely— it's the rare diabetes patient who can't exercise. So don't discard your workout clothes. Follow the example of these professional athletes, all of whom have diabetes but still managed to compete with the best and win. In baseball, there's Jackie Robinson, Ty Cobb, and Catfish Hunter. In football, Jonathan Hayes and Mike Pyle. And there are many others: Scott Verplank and Sherri Turner (golf), Bobby Clarke (hockey), Gene Horton (marathon running), Hamilton Richardson (tennis), and Bill Carlson (triathlon), to name but a few.

SOME CONCLUDING THOUGHTS

In this book, I've offered you a state-of-the-art method for using regular exercise to optimize both the quality and the quantity of your life. My advice has been based on what is currently known about exercise and diabetes. In years to come, far more will be learned about how diabetes patients, such as yourself, can benefit the most from an exercise rehabilitation program. But don't wait until then to begin a physically active lifestyle. Now is the time for you, in consultation with your doctor, to design your specific exercise plan from the prototype I've provided.

The sooner you begin a sensible exercise program, the sooner you'll reap the many rewards. Once you do get started, never forget that exercise should be fun. I've always enjoyed it thoroughly and have no doubt that with time you will, too.

Good luck! And the best of health to you.

Chapter 6
Prescription

❐ Have a detailed medical evaluation before you begin your exercise program and at regular intervals thereafter.
❐ Know the warning signs of an impending cardiac complication.
❐ Warm up and cool down adequately—allow a minimum of 5 minutes for each.
❐ Don't exercise in adverse climatic conditions, particularly without taking adequate precautions.
❐ Pay special attention to proper foot care.
❐ Memorize the symptoms of hypoglycemia. Know how to prevent it and what to do if you experience it.
❐ Know how to prevent late-onset hypoglycemia, which can occur 4 or more hours after exercise.

Appendix A

How to Take Your Pulse and Calculate Your Heart Rate

Y ou have two pulse points to choose from—the radial artery in your wrist or the carotid artery in your throat. Your radial artery is the preferred place because the reading there is usually more accurate.

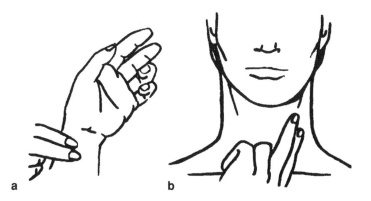

a   b

Figure A.1   Pulse points: a) radial artery, b) carotid artery. *Note.* From *ACSM Fitness Book* (p. 24) by The American College of Sports Medicine, 1992, Champaign, IL: Leisure Press. Copyright 1992 by The American College of Sports Medicine. Reprinted by permission.

Your two carotid arteries are located on either side of your windpipe. These arteries are large, and you should be able to locate them easily by gently pressing just to the right or left of your Adam's apple. But there are several things you must keep in mind. Don't press hard; press on only one carotid artery at a time; and do not press too near the jawbone. If you do any of these things your heart rate may slow down excessively and result in potentially harmful consequences, not to mention an inaccurate reading.

Taking your pulse is a three-step process. Here are instructions for taking a wrist pulse reading. Resort to your carotid artery only if you absolutely cannot locate the radial artery in your wrist.

1. *Locate the pulse in your wrist.* The hand of your wristwatch arm is the one you will use to monitor the pulse in your opposite wrist. Your "sensors" are the pads of your fingers, not your fingertips.

Place your index finger and middle finger at the base of the outer third of your wrist, the side on which your thumb is located. If you feel your wrist's tendons, you need to move your fingers further to the outside of your wrist. Do this incrementally, changing the location of your fingers by about a quarter of an inch until you finally locate a pulsation. Don't press too hard or you may obliterate your pulse. A light but firm pressure is all that is needed. You should be able to feel your pulse each time your heart beats, thus making your pulse rate equivalent to your heart rate.

2. *Count your pulse.* To determine your *resting heart rate*, count for 30 to 60 seconds. Your heart rate varies with your breathing; it slows down when you exhale and speeds up when you inhale. Thus if you count your pulse for shorter periods, you won't get a good average reading.

Taking a reading during exercise is different. Then your pulse rate is faster so a 10-second count is sufficient. If you're exercising in a stationary position—on a cycle ergometer, for example—you can count your pulse easily without stopping. However, if you're moving—such as walking or jogging—you'll need to stop, but not completely. Keep your legs moving while you take your pulse, which *you must do immediately*. If you wait for more than a second or two, your heart starts to slow down. This is true particularly if you are fit. If you count for longer than 10 seconds, you run the risk of greatly *underestimating* your heart rate.

When counting your pulse, count as "one" the first pulsation you feel *after* your watchhand hits a digit. Do *not* count as "one" any pulsation that occurs at the same time as the hand hits the digit.

Continue the count until your watch registers 10 seconds. If a pulsation occurs at the same time as the watchhand hits the 10-second point, count it, but none thereafter.

3. *Calculate your heart rate.* After you've counted your pulse for 10 seconds, multiply that number by 6 to get your heart rate (beats per minute). Here's a chart with the calculations already done for 10-second pulse counts of 12 through 31:

12 = 72	17 = 102	22 = 132	27 = 162
13 = 78	18 = 108	23 = 138	28 = 168
14 = 84	19 = 114	24 = 144	29 = 174
15 = 90	20 = 120	25 = 150	30 = 180
16 = 96	21 = 126	26 = 156	31 = 186

Appendix B

Hallmarks of a Comprehensive Medical Exam for Exercisers With Diabetes

Below, I describe what happens during a state-of-the-art medical exam in a facility that's fully equipped for sophisticated testing. Your checkup may not be as comprehensive if the equipment isn't available or if your medical history indicates that your case simply doesn't warrant it.

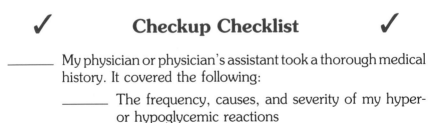

✓ Checkup Checklist ✓

_____ My physician or physician's assistant took a thorough medical history. It covered the following:

_____ The frequency, causes, and severity of my hyper- or hypoglycemic reactions

_____ For Type I diabetes patients and those with Type II diabetes who take insulin, the results of my self-monitored blood-glucose records

_____ Any problems I've had adhering to my prescribed therapeutic regimen

_____ Any adjustments I've made in my prescribed therapeutic regimen

_____ Any symptoms—such as chest pain or discomfort, loss of sensation in my feet, and visual disturbances—indicating I could be developing some of the long-term, chronic complications of diabetes

_____ Other existing medical ailments or conditions that I have

_____ My previous exercise history, if any

_____ My blood-sugar control was evaluated, including my glycosylated-hemoglobin measurement. This is essential because *my diabetes must be under reasonable control before I start my exercise program, especially if I have Type I diabetes.* If I'm taking too little insulin, exercise may exacerbate my Type I blood-sugar metabolism problems, increasing the possibility of hyperglycemia and ketoacidosis.

_____ I was given a thorough cardiovascular exam. It included the following:

_____ Blood-pressure measurement

_____ Monitoring of the pulses in my neck, arms, and legs

_____ Listening to my heart sounds and breathing

_____ A blood-lipid profile, which goes much further than a mere total cholesterol count

_____ A resting electrocardiogram (ECG)

_____ A treadmill exercise test if any of these conditions apply:

- I have any known or suspected cardiovascular disease.
- I have Type I diabetes and I'm over 30 years old.
- I've had Type I diabetes for more than 15 years.
- I have Type II diabetes and I'm over 35 years old.
- I have either Type I or Type II diabetes and also one or more other major risk factors for coronary artery disease—namely, high blood pressure, an

elevated cholesterol level, cigarette smoking, or a family history of coronary artery disease.

This is the precautionary approach strongly recommended by the American Diabetes Association and the American College of Sports Medicine.*

_____ I was given a thorough neurological evaluation, designed to identify any existing or developing autonomic or peripheral neurological disorders. This is crucial for all diabetes patients because autonomic neuropathy—that is, problems affecting nerves to organs such as the heart and blood vessels—can lead, during exercise, to an excessively slow heart rate; an inadequate rise, or even a fall, in systolic blood pressure; dizziness; fainting; quick exhaustion; an overheated body; or hypoglycemia. People with autonomic neuropathy may also be more prone to have silent rather than symptomatic heart disease and to have hypoglycemic unawareness.

People with peripheral neuropathy, which can cause pain or weakness in the legs, may find exercise more difficult. Another symptom—a loss of sensation in the feet and legs—predisposes a person to exercise injuries and ulcers.

_____ I was checked out for musculoskeletal problems. Special attention was paid to my feet to make sure there were no existing abnormalities that could worsen during exercise.

_____ I had an eye exam to detect preproliferative or proliferative retinopathy, both of which can get worse if I undertake inappropriate forms of exercise. If either condition was detected—or even suspected—I was given a more in-depth evaluation by an ophthalmologist.

---

*American College of Sports Medicine, *Guidelines for Exercise Testing and Prescription.* Philadelphia: Lea & Febiger, 1991 and American Diabetes Association. "Clinical Practice Recommendations, 1990-1991." Diabetes Care 14(1991):1-81.

FREQUENCY OF MEDICAL EXAMS AND SPECIFIC TESTS

Diabetes is a progressive disease that changes over time. New complications can develop and existing ones can worsen or, in some instances, get better or be made better by appropriate medical therapy.

Despite its health benefits, exercise does place a certain amount of stress on the body. If you exercise, it's particularly important for you to have periodic medical checkups. How often?

The frequency of follow-up medical exams depends on your type of diabetes, how well you're controlling your blood glucose, changes you've made to your prescribed therapeutic plan, and any chronic complications or other medical problems you have. Here are the recommendations of the American Diabetes Association about the frequency of physician visits:

- Any diabetes patient (Type I or Type II) being treated with insulin should have a checkup every 3 months, which should include a glycosylated-hemoglobin test. Otherwise, 6-month visits, which should also include this test, will suffice.
- In adults with diabetes, a fasting blood-lipid workup—including measurements of total cholesterol, HDL-cholesterol, and triglycerides—should be done annually; in children, every 2 years.
- Urine testing should be done annually. To detect the onset of diabetic nephropathy, it's critical to know the amount, if any, of protein leaving the body in urine, especially in adults or in anyone who has had diabetes for more than 5 years. If protein is found, more blood and kidney-function tests will be necessary.

SOURCE: American Diabetes Association. "Position Statement: Standards of Medical Care for Patients with Diabetes Mellitus." *Diabetes Care*, 13 (1990): 10-13.

Appendix C

Hypoglycemia Prevention Checklist

T o summarize all I've said about preventing hypoglycemia, the most common blood-sugar emergency for diabetes patients who exercise, I compiled the following checklist. I encourage you to post it in a prominent place and consult it often.

✓ Checklist for Preventing Hypoglycemia ✓

The best way to deal with the life-threatening condition of hypoglycemia is not to experience it at all. This checklist covers 10 of the most important factors that increase the risk of developing hypoglycemia. People with Type I diabetes, and those with Type II who are on insulin therapy or who are taking oral hypoglycemic agents, are at risk for hypoglycemia. If that includes you, post this checklist on your mental bulletin board. If you can place a checkmark next to each entry before every workout, you should never have to encounter hypoglycemia.

_____ I reduce my insulin or sulfonylurea dose before exercise, especially if the workout will be strenuous or longer than 1 hour, or if I'll be exercising when my injected insulin will be exerting its peak effect.

_____ I'm careful not to exercise within 60 minutes after an insulin injection, especially if the exercise involves the part of the body where the insulin was injected.

_____ I try to exercise 1 to 3 hours after eating a regularly scheduled meal or snack.

_____ I eat about 30 minutes after an insulin injection, not before the injection or only a few minutes afterward.

_____ I'm aware of the dangers of changing insulin sources. Human insulin has the most rapid onset and shortest duration of activity, whereas beef insulins have the slowest onset and the longest duration of activity.

_____ I'm aware of the consequences of changing insulin injection sites and make adjustments accordingly. The abdomen has the fastest rate of absorption, followed by my arms, thighs, and buttocks.

_____ I self-monitor my blood glucose before, during, and after exercise, particularly if the workout is strenuous and lasts longer than 1 hour.

_____ I eat or drink adequate amounts of carbohydrate before, during, and after exercise, particularly if my blood-glucose level is below 100 mg/dl or if the workout is strenuous and lasts longer than 1 hour.

_____ I begin an exercise program slowly and increase the intensity and duration gradually.

_____ I check with my doctor when starting or stopping a new medication to see if it may increase my risk for hypoglycemia.

Notes

CHAPTER 1

[1]Mazur, M. "Diabetes on Your Dial." *Diabetes Forecast* October 1989: 14-19.

CHAPTER 2

[1]Sushruta, S.C.S. *Vaidya Jadavaji Trikamji Acharia.* Bombay: Nirnyar Sagar Press, 1938.

[2]Allen, F.M., Stillman, E., and Fitz, R. "Total Dietary Regulation in the Treatment of Diabetes." In *Exercise*, edited by F.M. Allen, E. Stillman, and R. Fitz. New York: Rockefeller Institute, 1919.

[3]Lawrence, R.D. "The Effect of Exercise on Insulin Action in Diabetes." *British Medical Journal* 1 (1926): 648-650.

[4]Vranic, M., Wasserman, D., and Bukowieck, L. "Metabolic Implications of Exercise and Physical Fitness in Physiology and Diabetes." In *Diabetes Mellitus: Theory and Practice*, edited by H. Rifkin and D. Porte. New York: Elsevier, 1990: 198-219.

[5]Wallberg-Henriksson, H., et al. "Increased Peripheral Insulin Sensitivity and Muscle Mitochondrial Enzymes But Unchanged Blood Glucose Control in Type I Diabetics After Physical Training." *Diabetes* 31 (1982): 1044-1050.

[6]Zinman, B., Zuniga-Guajardo, S., and Kelly, D. "Comparison of the Acute and Long-Term Effects of Exercise on Glucose Control in Type I Diabetes." *Diabetes* 7 (1984): 515-519.

[7]Stratton, R., et al. "Improved Glycemic Control After Supervised 8-Week Exercise Program in Insulin-Dependent Diabetic Adolescents." *Diabetes Care* 10 (1987): 589-593.

[8]Ekoe, J.M. "Overview of Diabetes Mellitus and Exercise." *Medicine and Science in Sports and Exercise* 21 (1989): 353-355.

[9]Helmrich, P., et al. "Physical Activity and Reduced Occurrence of Non-Insulin-Dependent Diabetes Mellitus." *New England Journal of Medicine* 325 (1991): 147-152.

[10]Takekoshi, H., et al. "A 10-Year Follow-Up Study in NIDDM With or Without Exercise." In *Proceedings of the International Symposium on Epidemiology of Diabetes Mellitus*, edited by S. Vannasaeng, W. Nitiyanant, and S. Chandrapasert. Bangkok (1987): 149-152.

[11]Bogardus, C., et al. "Effects of Physical Training and Diet Therapy on Carbohydrate Metabolism in Patients with Glucose Intolerance and Non-Insulin-Dependent Diabetes Mellitus." *Diabetes* 33 (1984): 311-318.

[12]National Institutes of Health. "Consensus Development Conference on Diet and Exercise in Non-Insulin-Dependent Diabetes Mellitus." *Diabetes Care* 10 (1987): 639-644.

[13]Brownell, K.D. "Weight Management and Body Composition." In *Resource Manual for Guidelines for Exercise Testing and Prescription*, edited by S.N. Blair et al. Philadelphia: Lea & Febiger, 1988: 355-361.

[14]King, A., et al. "Diet Versus Exercise in Weight Maintenance: The Effects of Minimal Intervention Strategies on Long-Term Outcomes in Men." *Archives of Internal Medicine* 149 (1989): 2741-2746.

[15]Cunningham, L.N. "Commentary: Comparison of the Acute and Long-Term Effects of Exercise on Glucose Control in Type I Diabetes." *Diabetes Spectrum* 1 (1988): 224-225.

[16]American Diabetes Association. "Position Statement: Blood Glucose Control in Diabetes." *Diabetes Care* 13 (1990): 16-17.

[17]Powell, K.E., et al. "Physical Activity and the Incidence of Coronary Heart Disease." *Annual Review of Public Health* 8 (1987): 253-287.

[18]Berlin, G.A., and Colditz, G.A. "A Meta-Analysis of Physical Activity in the Prevention of Coronary Heart Disease." *American Journal of Epidemiology* 132 (1990): 612-628.

[19]Fletcher, G.F., et al. "AHA Medical/Scientific Statement on Exercise." *Circulation* 86 (1992): 340-344.

CHAPTER 3

[1]Miller, W.J., Sherman, W.M., and Ivy, J.L. "Effect of Strength Training on Glucose Tolerance and Post-Glucose Insulin Response." *Medicine and Science in Sports and Exercise* 16 (1984): 539-543.

[2]Institute for Aerobics Research. *The Strength Connection*. Dallas: Institute for Aerobics Research, 1990.

³American College of Sports Medicine. "Position Stand: The Recommended Quantity and Quality of Exercise for Developing and Maintaining Cardiorespiratory and Muscular Fitness in Healthy Adults." *Medicine and Science in Sports and Exercise* 22 (1990): 265-274.

⁴Gordon, N.F., and Gibbons, L.W. *The Cooper Clinic Cardiac Rehabilitation Program.* New York: Simon & Schuster, 1990.

⁵Cooper, K.H. *Aerobics.* New York: Bantam Books, 1968.

⁶Blair, S.N., et al. "Exercise and Fitness in Childhood: Implications for a Lifetime of Health." In *Perspective in Exercise Science and Sports Medicine 2: Youth, Exercise and Sport*, edited by C.V. Gisolfi and D.R. Lamb. Indianapolis: Benchmark Press, 1989: 401-430.

⁷American Heart Association. "Exercise Standards: A Statement for Health Professionals from the American Heart Association." *Circulation* 82 (1990): 2286-2322.

⁸Haskell, W.L., Montoye, H.J., and Orenstein, D. "Physical Activity and Exercise to Achieve Health-Related Physical Fitness Components." *Public Health Reports* 100 (1985): 202-212.

⁹Blair, S.N. *Living with Exercise.* Dallas: American Health Publishing Co., 1991.

¹⁰American Diabetes Association. "Technical Review: Exercise and NIDDM." *Diabetes Care* 14 (1991): 52-56.

¹¹DeBusk, R.F., et al. "Training Effects of Long Versus Short Bouts of Exercise in Healthy Subjects." *American Journal of Cardiology* 65 (1990): 1010-1013.

¹²American Diabetes Association. "Position Statement: Diabetes Mellitus and Exercise." *Diabetes Care* 14 (1991): 36-37.

¹³Mitchell, Y.H., et al. "Hyperglycemia After Intense Exercise in IDDM Subjects During Continuous Subcutaneous Insulin Infusion." *Diabetes Care* 11 (1988): 311-317.

¹⁴Borg, G.A. "Psychophysical Bases of Perceived Exertion." *Medicine and Science in Sports and Exercise* 14 (1982): 377-387.

¹⁵Rippe, J.M., et al. "Walking for Health and Fitness." *Journal of the American Medical Association* 259 (1988): 2720-2724.

¹⁶Thomas, T.R., and Londeree, B.R. "Energy Cost During Prolonged Walking Vs. Jogging Exercise." *Physician and Sportsmedicine* 17 (1989): 93-102.

CHAPTER 4

¹Cooper, K.H. *The Aerobics Program for Total Well-Being.* New York: Bantam Books, 1982.

²Gwinup, G. "Weight Loss Without Dietary Restriction: Efficacy of Different Forms of Aerobic Exercise." *American Journal of Sports Medicine* 15 (1987): 275-279.

³Cooper, K.H. *Overcoming Hypertension.* New York: Bantam Books, 1990.

[4]DeBenedette, V. "Stair Machines: The Truth About This Fitness Fad." *Physician and Sportsmedicine* 18 (1990): 131-134.

[5]Gordon, N.F., et al. "Effects of Rest Interval Duration on Cardiorespiratory Responses to Hydraulic Resistance Circuit Training." *Journal of Cardiopulmonary Rehabilitation* 9 (1989): 325-330.

[6]Paffenbarger, Jr., R.S., et al. "Physical Activity, All-Cause Mortality, and Longevity in College Alumni." *New England Journal of Medicine* 314 (1986): 605-613.

[7]Coyle, E.F. "Detraining and Retension of Training-Induced Adaptations." In *Resource Manual for Guidelines for Exercise Testing and Prescription*, edited by S.N. Blair et al. Philadelphia: Lea & Febiger, 1988: 83-89.

CHAPTER 5

[1]American Diabetes Association. "Consensus Statement: Self-Monitoring of Blood Glucose." *Diabetes Care* 13 (1990): 41-46.

[2]Stratton, R., Wilson, D.P., and Endres, R.K. "Acute Glycemic Effects of Exercise in Adolescents with Insulin-Dependent Diabetes Mellitus." *Physician and Sportsmedicine* 16 (1988): 150-157.

[3]Mazur, M. "Lady With a Drive." *Diabetes Forecast* August 1989: 29-31.

[4]Trovati, M., et al. "Postprandial Exercise in Type I Diabetic Patients on Multiple Daily Insulin Injection Regimen." *Diabetes Care* 11 (1988): 107-110.

[5]Ruegemer, J.J., et al. "Differences Between Pre-Breakfast and Late Afternoon Glycemic Responses to Exercise in IDDM Patients." *Diabetes Care* 13 (1990): 104-110.

[6]Cryer, P.E., et al. "Hypoglycemia in IDDM." *Diabetes* 38 (1989): 1193-1199.

[7]Horton, E.S. "Exercise and Diabetes Mellitus." In *The Medical Clinics of North America*, edited by R.A. Rizza and D.A. Greene. Philadelphia: W.B. Saunders Co., Vol. 72, No. 6, 1988.

[8]Kemmer, F.W., et al. "Prevention of Exercise Induced Hypoglycemia in Diabetes Mellitus." *Diabetes* 35 (1986): 963-967.

[9]Coleman, E. "Sports Drink Update." *Gatorade Sports Science Exchange* 1; 5 (1988).

[10]Davis, J.M., et al. "Fluid Availability of Sports Drinks Differing in Carbohydrate Type and Concentration." *American Journal of Clinical Nutrition* 51 (1990): 1054-1057.

[11]Franz, M.J., and Norstrom, J. *Diabetes: Actively Staying Healthy.* Wayzata, MN: DCI Publishing, 1990.

CHAPTER 6

[1]American Diabetes Association. "Position Statement: Diabetes Mellitus and Exercise." *Diabetes Care* 13 (1990): 804-805.

[2]Hollingsworth, D.R., and Moore, T.R. "Postprandial Walking Exercise in Pregnant Insulin-Dependent (Type I) Diabetic Women: Reduction of Plasma Lipid Levels but Absence of a Significant Effect on Glycemic Control." *American Journal of Obstetrics and Gynecology* 157 (1987): 1359-1363.

[3]Second International Workshop-Conference on Gestational Diabetes Mellitus. "Summary and Recommendations of the Second International Workshop-Conference on Gestational Diabetes Mellitus." *Diabetes* 34 (1985): 123-126.

[4]Cooper, K.H., and Cooper, M. *The New Aerobics for Women*. New York: Bantam Books, 1988.

[5]Cooper, K.H. *Running Without Fear*. New York: M. Evans & Co., 1985.

[6]Cooper, K.H. *The Aerobics Program for Total Well-Being*. New York: Bantam Books, 1982.

[7]Bild, D.E., et al. "Lower-Extremity Amputation in People with Diabetes." *Diabetes* 12 (1989): 24-31.

[8]MacDonald, M.J. "Postexercise Late-Onset Hypoglycemia in Insulin-Dependent Diabetes Patients." *Diabetes Care* 10 (1987): 584-588.

[9]Kemmer, F.W., et al. "Exercise-Induced Fall of Blood Glucose in Insulin-Treated Diabetics Unrelated to Alteration of Insulin Mobilization." *Diabetes* 28 (1979): 1131-1137.

Index